Polycystic Ovary Syndrome
Novel Insights into Causes and Therapy

Frontiers of Hormone Research

Vol. 40

Series Editor

Ashley B. Grossman Oxford

Polycystic Ovary Syndrome

Novel Insights into Causes and Therapy

Volume Editors

Djuro Macut Belgrade

Marija Pfeifer Ljubljana

Bulent Okan Yildiz Ankara

Evanthia Diamanti-Kandarakis Athens

11 figures, 3 in color, and 10 tables, 2013

KARGER Basel · Freiburg · Paris · London · New York · New Delhi · Bangkok · Beijing · Tokyo · Kuala Lumpur · Singapore · Sydney

Djuro Macut, MD, PhD
Clinic for Endocrinology, Diabetes and Metabolic Diseases
Faculty of Medicine
University of Belgrade
Belgrade, Serbia

Bulent Okan Yildiz, MD
Endocrinology and Metabolism Unit
Department of Internal Medicine
Hacettepe University School of Medicine
Ankara, Turkey

Marija Pfeifer, MD, PhD
Department of Endocrinology, Diabetes and Metabolic Diseases
University Medical Centre Ljubljana
Ljubljana, Slovenia

Evanthia Diamanti-Kandarakis, MD, PhD
Endocrine Unit
Third Department of Internal Medicine
Medical School
National and Kapodistrian University of Athens
Athens, Greece

Library of Congress Cataloging-in-Publication Data

Polycystic ovary syndrome: novel insights into causes and therapy / volume editors,
Djuro Macut ... [et al.].
p. ; cm. -- (Frontiers of hormone research, ISSN 0301-3073; v. 40)
Includes bibliographical references and indexes.
ISBN 978-3-318-02238-4 (hard cover: alk. paper) -- ISBN 978-3-318-02239-1 (electronic version)
I. Macut, Djuro. II. Series: Frontiers of hormone research; v. 40. 0301-3073
[DNLM: 1. Polycystic Ovary Syndrome--etiology. 2. Metabolic Syndrome X--complications.
3. Polycystic Ovary Syndrome--therapy. W1 FR946F v.40 2013 / WP 320]

618.1'1--dc23

2012033313

Bibliographic Indices. This publication is listed in bibliographic services, including Current Contents® and PubMed/MEDLINE.

www.karger.com
Printed in Switzerland on acid-free and non-aging paper (ISO 9706) by Reinhardt Druck, Basel
ISSN 0301–3073
e-ISSN 1662–3762
ISBN 978–3–318–02238–4
e-ISBN 978–3–318–02239–1

Contents

Foreword

Polycystic ovarian disease is a worldwide disorder which is seen in all populations and ethnic groups, although its manifestations may vary according to ethnicity. Such patients may present with irregular menses, hirsuties, acne or other signs of androgen excess, or sometimes infertility. Unfortunately, this common and distressing condition is often either ignored or dismissed by many clinicians as essentially 'cosmetic', and indeed often its manifestations may be mild and of little consequence. However, in many women it causes considerable concern and distress, and the hirsuties in particular can cause dramatic concern with regard to body image and feelings of femininity and attractiveness. Furthermore, there is now increasing evidence that there are long-term implications of polycystic ovarian disease over and beyond any short-term cosmetic concerns: the development of type 2 diabetes and the metabolic syndrome are clearly of major significance. But why is this condition so common, especially as it may compromise reproductive fitness in the reproductive years? Are there important genetic aspects, how can we best manage these patients, how is it related to the later development of the metabolic syndrome, and what are the optimal therapies currently and on the horizon? It should also be remembered that the condition is sometimes a secondary phenomenon to other disease states. These are the questions which Marija Pfeifer and her colleagues have addressed in this important volume based on a symposium held in 2012, where an international panel of experts gathered to try and make sense of the increasing data amassed over the past few years. We hope that by bringing together these contributions from such an international array of clinicians and scientists we can make such current knowledge available to all that may come across and treat this fascinating condition, and optimize the treatment for each and every patient.

Ashley B. Grossman, Oxford

Preface

The most frequent disorder affecting women of reproductive age is polycystic ovary syndrome (PCOS). PCOS has long been a field surrounded by considerable uncertainty as regards its etiology and pathogenesis, identification of its manifestations within the various disciplines of medicine, as well concerning the decision as to optimal treatment modalities. In the early years, the understanding of this syndrome was based on recognizing its clinical appearance in the presence of ovarian morphology. However, recently substantial advances have been made in knowledge pertaining to the complex genetic, biochemical, metabolic, cardiovascular, and reproductive issues associated with PCOS, with the result that today an integrative approach is being established in the understanding and management of the syndrome.

Insight into the specific endocrine and metabolic causes and consequences still remains the clinical cornerstone for full understanding of the syndrome and for further future development. Such advancement of our knowledge is absolutely essential since, in the absence of better therapeutic options to resolve its key metabolic and biochemical derangements, women with PCOS have for long been faced with the same problems and prospects as the majority of patients suffering from obesity and metabolic syndrome. Meanwhile, since the acronym PCOS still points to the ovary as the most prominent marker of the syndrome, the time may have come for general reappraisal of the syndrome – and its naming! – so as to adopt a far more global approach to its confrontation and more metabolic-oriented methods for its resolution.

This book presents a broad overview of recent developments in identifying the phenotypic expression of women with PCOS, this having been greatly clarified via recent clinical efforts to specifically define the syndrome, resulting in a completely new recognition of its phenotypic variability. The various parts of the volume are devoted to acquainting the reader with the metabolic and cardiovascular consequences of the syndrome, advances made in dealing with secondary forms of PCOS-like syndromes, as well as specific therapies of clinical symptoms and signs and the outcomes of these therapies. Additionally incorporated are a number of 'hot topics' related to genetic developments, endothelial causes leading to the unfavorable outcomes, and novelties in therapeutic approaches oriented to better resolution of metabolic and reproductive consequences.

The multiple aspects of the PCOS have been addressed in this comprehensive work by leading experts in the field and their teams. This reflects the editors' intention not only to assemble a volume for the reader's easy access to specifics regarding the characteristics and consequences of this syndrome, but also to offer a substantial body of critical scientific knowledge, this divided into twelve chapters. Thanks to the invaluable contributions of the authors, the present work succeeds in proposing a contemporary endocrine overview on PCOS, and we hope with a distinctive European flavor.

We would like to sincerely thank the authors for their expert submissions and their highly constructive contributions throughout the compilation of the book. We also take this opportunity to gratefully acknowledge the noble endeavors of the leading experts to develop European endocrine study groups on PCOS that focus not only on reproductive endocrine issues per se but also on the ongoing effort for integration of endocrinology with related fields of medicine.

Djuro Macut, Belgrade
Marija Pfeifer, Ljubljana
Bulent Okan Yildiz, Ankara
Evanthia Diamanti-Kandarakis, Athens

Macut D, Pfeifer M, Yildiz BO, Diamanti-Kandarakis E (eds): Polycystic Ovary Syndrome. Novel Insights into Causes and Therapy. Front Horm Res. Basel, Karger, 2013, vol 40, pp 1–21

Polycystic Ovary Syndrome: Definitions, Phenotypes and Diagnostic Approach

Sarantis Livadas · Evanthia Diamanti-Kandarakis

Endocrine Unit, Third Department of Internal Medicine, Medical School, National and Kapodistrian University of Athens, Athens, Greece

Abstract

Polycystic ovary syndrome (PCOS) constitutes a continuum spectrum of symptoms starting from the early prepubertal years and continuing after menopause. The phenotypic expression varies through time, depending on several internal (e.g. ovarian/adrenal steroidogenesis, insulin resistance) and external factors (e.g. quality and quantity of food, exercise). Moreover, the emergence of new definitions with the use of ovarian morphology, besides chronic anovulation and hyperandrogenism, as diagnostic criteria, increased the phenotypic variety of PCOS presentation. In this review, the clinician is provided with useful information regarding grey zones in assessing anovulation, hyperandrogenism, ovarian morphology and the difficulties in differential diagnosis of PCOS. Furthermore, the lack of substantial data characterizing metabolic/hormonal profile and the potential cardiovascular risk in newer PCOS phenotypes, as well as the absence of longitudinal data questioning a possible shift from one phenotype to another are underlined. These notions indicate that despite the initial presentation of a patient with PCOS, close follow-up and therapeutic interventions aiming to reduce long-term cardiovascular risk are warranted.

Polycystic ovary syndrome (PCOS) constitutes the most common endocrinopathy of women of reproductive age. It has gained a great deal of public attention over the last few decades, as this is reflected in over 1,500,000 Internet sites dedicated to the syndrome. However, although widespread, PCOS is a very complex endocrine condition, making its diagnosis a difficult and challenging task in everyday clinical practice. These difficulties in diagnosis, as well as the heterogeneity of the disease and its nebulous nature, were made evident from the very first description of PCOS by Stein and Leventhal. Specifically, among the 7 women described in the original report, a variety of clinical symptoms were observed, such as obesity, hirsutism, acne, and amenorrhea, all of which were associated with enlarged bilateral polycystic ovaries. These distinctive features, displaying a varying degree of expression in each case, emphasize the phenotypic variability of PCOS and, in fact, explain why it is defined as a syndrome and not a disease.

A syndrome is a cluster of symptoms, which cannot be explained under the prism of a common etiologic factor or a unifying pathophysiological pathway. Furthermore, the fact that hormones act in almost all tissues but at a different rate, this depending on their receptor function and post-receptor signaling, accounts to a considerable degree for the variety of clinical expression observed in hormonal disorders and metabolic aberrations. This situation is further complicated in PCOS in which more than one hormone secretion is modified. More specifically, women with PCOS manifest hyperandrogenemia, hyperinsulinemia, and hypothalamic-pituitary-ovarian axis aberrations, as well as adipose tissue dysfunctional adipokine secretion, all of which interact in different tissues (fat, liver, muscle and ovaries), thus leading to a variety of phenotypes. Due to these difficulties, the definition of PCOS has been a matter of constant debate, and the different combinations of symptoms and signs have through the years resulted in significant variations of diagnosis and management between different groups.

Definitions and Phenotypes

In 1990, the publication of strict National Institutes of Health (NIH) criteria, which make obligatory for the diagnosis the concomitant presence of anovulation and hyperandrogenemia on either the biochemical or the clinical level (hirsutism/acne), underscored the fact that PCOS is a metabolic/reproductive disorder. However, since the common perception was that polycystic morphology (PCOM) was a characteristic finding in these women, the absence of inclusion of ovarian PCOM gave rise to a great many discrepancies on clinical grounds. Although excellent studies have since clearly demonstrated that polycystic ovarian morphology on ultrasound may be found in about 20–30% of normally ovulating, but not hyperandrogenemic women, for a significant number of physicians (especially Europeans), this distinction was mandatory for the diagnosis. This fallacy led in 2004 (Rotterdam) to the formulation of new diagnostic criteria whereby the presence of all these three factors (chronic anovulation, hyperandrogenism, and polycystic ovaries on ultrasonography) was evaluated and PCOS was diagnosed in the presence of two of the three diagnostic criteria. Using the possible combinations of these criteria, four different phenotypes of PCOS are now identified:

- Type A: hyperandrogenism, chronic anovulation and polycystic ovaries.
- Type B: hyperandrogenism and chronic anovulation.
- Type C: hyperandrogenism and polycystic ovaries.
- Type D: chronic anovulation and polycystic ovaries.

These different phenotypes are illustrated in figure 1.

The Rotterdam criteria do not delineate the essential features of PCOS, since they identify PCOM as being equivalent to chronic anovulation and hyperandrogenism

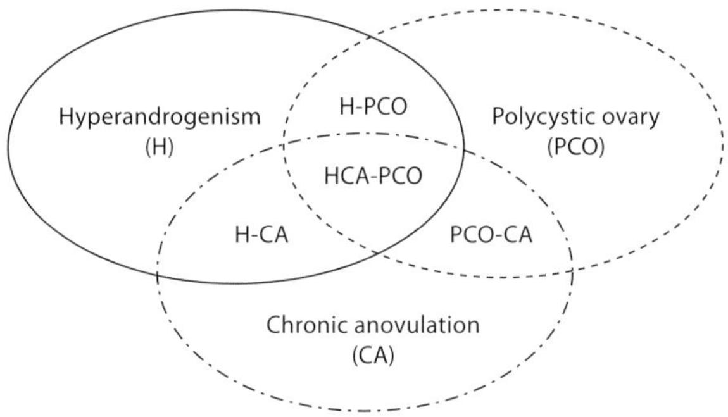

Fig. 1. The different phenotypes in PCOS. Type A: hyperandrogenism, chronic anovulation and polycystic ovaries; type B: hyperandrogenism and chronic anovulation; type C: hyperandrogenism and polycystic ovaries; type D: chronic anovulation and polycystic ovaries.

as regards diagnosis. These criteria, however, laid emphasis on the fact that PCOS could manifest via a spectrum of symptoms, thus implying that it may be diagnosed in the absence of androgen excess. Many authorities in the field questioned this position, and in 2006 the Androgen Excess Society (AES) pointed out that PCOS is basically a hyperandrogenic disorder, and that the existence of hirsutism/acne and/or hyperandrogenemia constitutes a sine qua non for PCOS diagnosis. The second criterion essential for the diagnosis according to the AES is either anovulation or polycystic ovarian morphology. These criteria were further consolidated in 2009 by the Androgen Excess and PCOS Society Task Force statement. All definitions mentioned above are presented in table 1. However, despite the presence of these several definitions, PCOS is still a diagnosis of exclusion of other androgenic entities. Furthermore, none of these definitions has been verified in adolescents in whom anovulation, PCOM, and hyperandrogenism usually occur for a temporary period [1, 2].

Most importantly, it should be stated that these various definitions are products of consensus statements, namely the majority opinion, and not the robust and solid findings of clinical trial evidence. This disadvantage is reflected in the vague nature of the definitions and in the lack of compliance of all medical authorities with these definitions. Moreover, the array of various definitions available in the literature has increased confusion regarding PCOS diagnosis, especially among different specialties. This situation was clearly illustrated in a study conducted by Cussons et al. [3] involving 138 endocrinologists and 172 gynecologists among whom different criteria were used for diagnosis. Specifically, 70% of endocrinologists versus half of the gynecologists considered menstrual irregularity as an essential criterion, whereas 60% of the gynecology group versus 14% of endocrinologists judged polycystic ovaries on ultrasound as an essential tool for PCOS diagnosis. Furthermore, although this study was carried out in 2005, less than 15% of gynecologists would use either the NIH or

Table 1. Definitions of PCOS

Definition/year	Diagnostic criteria[1]
NIH/1990	Requires the simultaneous presence of: 1. Hyperandrogenism (clinical and/or biochemical) 2. Ovarian dysfunction
Rotterdam (ESHRE/ASRM)/2003	Requires the presence of at least two criteria: 1. Hyperandrogenism (clinical and/or biochemical) 2. Ovulatory dysfunction 3. Polycystic ovarian morphology[2]
AES/2006	Requires the presence of hyperandrogenism (clinical and/or biochemical) and either: 1. Ovulatory dysfunction 2. Polycystic ovarian morphology[2]
Androgen Excess and PCOS Society/2009	Requires the simultaneous presence of: 1. Hyperandrogenism (clinical and/or biochemical) 2. Ovarian dysfunction (ovulatory dysfunction and/or polycystic ovarian morphology[2])

[1] It is important to state that as well as being well established by all the diagnostic criteria available PCOS diagnosis is an exclusion diagnosis of other disorders, such as NC-CAH, Cushing syndrome, acromegaly, hyperprolactinemia, hypothyroidism, premature ovarian failure, virilizing adrenal or ovarian neoplasm and a drug-related condition.
[2] The ultrasound definition of polycystic ovarian morphology is the presence of ≥12 follicles with a 2- to 9-mm diameter on the ovary. An ovarian volume >10 ml is also suggestive. Only one ovary consistent with polycystic ovarian morphology is sufficient for the diagnosis.
ESHRE = European Society for Human Reproduction and Embryology; ASRM = American Society for Reproductive Medicine.

Rotterdam criteria for diagnosis. Although these percentages were higher, they were also not acceptable among endocrinologists (about 40%). These data demonstrate the existing broad discrepancy in PCOS diagnosis, which is reflected in everyday practice. The aim of this review is to provide an overview of the current knowledge concerning the varying phenotypic expression of PCOS according to current definitions as well as a proposal as to which could be the ideal diagnostic approach [3].

Prevalence of Phenotypes Based on Different Criteria

PCOS is considered to be the most common endocrine disorder in women of reproductive age. However, the actual prevalence of PCOS in the community is the subject of a continuing debate due to the specific sampling methodology used in each of the various studies as well as study design limitations. Nevertheless, PCOS prevalence based on the NIH criteria is estimated to be about 6–8% in women of Caucasian origin, although with the implementation of the Rotterdam criteria, the prevalence increased to 15–25%, while the use of AES recommendations put PCOS prevalence at about 10–15%. These findings strongly suggest that a thorough understanding of PCOS pathophysiology and its association with reproductive and metabolic disturbances is essential for any physician addressing women's health, since the very large number of patients he/she will encounter will make it more than evident that this concerns a highly multifaceted syndrome [4, 5].

PCOS Phenotypes through Life Cycle

The development of PCOS has been associated with a sequence of events affecting fetal life and the programming of endocrine axes, especially carbohydrate metabolism and adrenals secretion. Indeed, girls born small for gestational age or large for gestational age, this being an indirect index of exposure to stressful intrauterine conditions, manifest a high incidence of PCOS in adolescence. Furthermore, in girls with early adrenal androgen secretion clinically disclosed as premature pubarche, several components of PCOS have been found, such as insulin resistance and visceral adiposity, in comparison to their normal peers. In addition, an increased proportion of these girls develop PCOS in adolescence, indicating a common pathogenetic link between these two nosologic entities. Also most interestingly, girls born small for gestational age who develop premature adrenarche later on have a significantly higher tendency to develop full-blown PCOS in adulthood compared to other girls who express only one of these two conditions. This observation suggests that exposure of a female to harmful events during fetal life and the peripubertal period may considerably affect her metabolic, hormonal, and reproductive phenotype [6].

With regard to post-menopause, there are strong indications that exposure to numerous cardiovascular (CV) risk factors that have set in as from adolescence has a profound impact on mortality by multiplying post-menopause CV incidents. Although solid evidence is still lacking, available data point to higher rates of CV disease in women with a history of PCOS compared to age- and BMI-matched peers. However, it should be emphasized that these data were obtained from the evaluation of women strictly in accordance with the NIH criteria and not from those with PCOS diagnosis according to the Rotterdam criteria [7].

Common Problems with Respect to Criteria Used for PCOS Classification

Based on the currently used definitions, four different phenotypes have been established for PCOS classification, as illustrated in figure 1. It remains under investigation whether the spectrum of phenotypes reflects differences in the severity of the syndrome and its long-term complications. These issues have not as yet been clearly elucidated and conflicting data have been reported. The reason for this discordance is the heterogeneity of the syndrome, the different techniques applied in the several studies, and the lack of accuracy and reliability that is apparent in the evaluation of PCOS subjects. We will illustrate and underline these differences with the aim of constructing uniform diagnostic criteria for the diagnosis of PCOS within the range of the different phenotypes.

Androgens

Hyperandrogenemia constitutes one of the cardinal features of PCOS and, indeed, in a significant number of patients (60–80%) elevated circulating androgen levels have been disclosed. However, there are several basic points that the clinician should bear in mind regarding androgens and PCOS. First of all, circulating levels of androgens in women of reproductive age reflect both ovarian and adrenal production. Specifically, ovaries and adrenals contribute equally (50%) to total testosterone and androstenedione levels, whereas dehydroepiandrosterone sulfate (DHEAS) values are almost exclusively produced by the adrenals. This information is of basic clinical importance since basal androgen measurement may directly guide diagnosis to an adrenal source of hyperandrogenemia. Nevertheless, age also affects androgen levels, data providing evidence that there is a gradual fall through time. Furthermore, it must be emphasized that androgenic activity is not similar for all androgens. Specifically, dehydroepiandrosterone exerts the lower biological action, whereas testosterone is the most potent circulating androgen in women.

An as yet unresolved issue with respect to hyperandrogenemia in PCOS is: which is the best method for androgen assessment and especially testosterone? The vast majority of assays have been designed for testosterone estimation in males in whom normal values are ten times higher than in women. This methodological problem is reflected in the great variation of testosterone values among different assays employed in females. Although equilibrium dialysis and tandem mass spectrometry are considered the gold standard for testosterone estimation, they are very expensive and are limited to a certain number of laboratories, this making their use inappropriate on clinical basis. Since RIAs are not appropriate for measuring androgens in women due to their low diagnostic yield, immunoassay after extraction and chromatography is preferred as a more practicable and cheaper solution. However, the lack of an assay designed for the low testosterone concentrations found in women is a major limitation. To overcome this difficulty, the lab needs to introduce its own normal standards, also given the fact that there are national and regional differences of testosterone levels among different populations.

Another ongoing debate is whether total or free testosterone (FT) should be evaluated. It must be underlined that only 1–2% of testosterone circulates in its free and biologically active form, while the rest is bound tightly to SHBG (65%) and weakly to albumin (33%). Consequently, alteration of albumin levels or the existence of any factor modifying SHBG will affect total testosterone levels. Hyperinsulinemia and obesity, two common factors in PCOS, will decrease SHBG, and glucocorticoids and growth hormone exert the same effect. By contrast, thyroxine and estrogen will increase SHBG, this being one of the mechanisms of the therapeutic effects of oral contraceptives in PCOS. In order to overcome this difficulty, the use of the ratio of total testosterone to SHBG, namely the 'free androgen index' or FAI (FAI: the ratio of total testosterone to SHBG multiplied by 100), has been introduced as an index of bioavailable testosterone. However, this index has not been widely accepted as yet on clinical grounds, although several studies have shown a better correlation with PCOS features than total or FT values.

Nevertheless, the Androgen Excess Society and Endocrine Society have suggested that the measurement of FT concentration using high-quality and sensitive assays is the most useful test to detect hyperandrogenemia in PCOS. FT circulating levels reflect both the degree of ovarian and adrenal testosterone production as well as the proportion of testosterone bound to SHBG. Accordingly, in PCOS where androgen excess and inhibited SHBG hepatic production coexist, FT concentrations can be found elevated, even in the cases of patients with total testosterone levels in the normal range. In fact, several studies have found hyperandrogenemia with FT evaluation in about 60% of women with PCOS, whereas the analogous values for total testosterone were less than 50% [8].

The issue of which other androgens should be evaluated is still a matter of debate. There are data obtained from large studies showing that in about 30% of PCOS, only androstenedione levels are elevated and, furthermore, that these women exhibit a more 'severe' form of PCOS as regards metabolic profile. In addition, in 10% of women with PCOS only DHEAS levels are elevated, and in these cases a thorough evaluation via Synacthen test and even CYP21 genotyping is needed to exclude non-classical congenital adrenal hyperplasia (NC-CAH). However, the combined measurement of FT, total testosterone, and DHEAS has a higher sensitivity of 75% in distinguishing hyperandrogenemia in women with PCOS, versus normal population.

Another aspect that should be discussed is the impact of the specific day of menstrual cycle when blood sampling is carried out on androgens values. In general, the recommendation is that androgens be evaluated during the ovulatory phase, and especially on the first 3–5 days of menstruation, given that a 20–30% rise in both total and free testosterone takes place prior to the LH surge, namely between the 7th and 10th day of a normal ovulatory circle. Since many women visit their doctors during amenorrheic or oligomenorrheic periods, it is not easy to assess androgen levels that can best be measured during spontaneous menstruation.

Many clinicians thus suggest the induction of withdrawal bleeding with the use of progesterone with the aim of overcoming this difficulty. However, as our group has recently shown, it is far more useful to evaluate progesterone levels and, if they are suggestive of anovulation (levels <3 ng/ml) [9.54 nmol/l] to proceed the next day to androgen evaluation. The results obtained with this technique are similar to those obtained with the induction of withdrawal bleeding, enabling the assessment of androgens in a faster and much more effective way [9]. Finally, we should keep in mind that a spontaneous ovulation is capable of restoring androgen levels to normal range in a woman with PCOS despite the fact that hyperandrogenemia has been identified during anovulatory cycles.

In conclusion, although hyperandrogenemia is a sine qua non in PCOS diagnosis, there are still plenty of questions which have not been answered yet, namely: (a) which androgen(s) should be measured; (b) how often; (c) which are the normal androgen levels in women, and (d) which analytical techniques should be employed.

Hirsutism

Hirsutism is defined as excessive terminal hair growth that takes on a male pattern distribution. In order to better understand the phenomenon of hirsutism, some background information is needed. Hairs cover the entire surface of the human body, with the exception of the lips, palms of the hands, and soles of the feet. Hair type can be subdivided into three categories, asexual, ambo-sexual and sexual, depending on the effects of androgens. Asexual hair is localized in the eyebrows, the eyelashes, and the lateral and occipital scalp and is insensitive to androgens levels, whereas ambo-sexual hair is restricted to the pubis and axilla as well as the lower arms and legs, and is sensitive to low androgens levels. Sexual hair is that found on the chin, face, chest, abdomen, back, thighs, and upper arms, with high levels of circulating androgens being needed to generate its production. Accordingly, in PCOS the detection of increased hair in these areas, which is termed hirsutism, is suggestive of hyperandrogenism.

Although hirsutism constitutes the most common clinical manifestation of hyperandrogenism (60–70%) in women with PCOS, the estimation of its degree is still controversial. Several methods exist for the objective assessment of hair growth, such as the weighing of the hairs, the measurement of the outer diameter of either plucked or clipped hairs, the determination of hair density or the 'vellus index', etc. However, these techniques are costly and time-consuming and are, on the whole, not widely employed in the evaluation of PCOS. In contrast, in clinical practice excessive hair growth in women is generally quantified with the use of the Ferriman-Gallwey scoring system (FG). This system grades terminal hair growth on a scale from 0 to 4 on eleven anatomical sites and uses the sum of nine areas to generate an overall hirsutism score. Scores of ≥8 or ≥5 have been commonly accepted as abnormal, but this system has several disadvantages. It is highly subjective, and studies have shown as much as a 10-point variation between researchers evaluating the same patient.

Furthermore, as the FG score reflects the total score, hair growth on arms or legs is considered equivalent to hair growth on the face or chest, although these areas reflect different sensitivity to androgens, as explained above. In addition, age and ethnicity significantly influence hair growth due to variances in 5 α-reductase activity, so that different normal values should be expected among different populations and age groups, although precise determination of these has not as yet been established. Finally, the evaluation of certain areas (e.g. chest, thighs) causes discomfort in the patients, especially in the case of a woman being examined by a male examiner. Recently, a modified FG score was tried out assessing only chin and abdomen. This showed a good correlation with the total FG score and gave indication of being a promising approach, although it requires further verification from other research groups [10].

Anovulation

In 1990, the anovulatory process was pinpointed as being a chief manifestation of PCOS. Menstrual irregularity in women with PCOS occurs due to anovulation, and menstrual disturbances usually present in the form of oligo-amenorrhea (fewer than six to eight episodes of menstrual bleeding per year or menses that occur at intervals greater than 35 days). The medical definition of chronic anovulation in PCOS is based: (a) on the exclusion of other causes of anovulation (e.g. hyperprolactinemia, hypothyroidism, etc.), and (b) on the measurement of progesterone values 8–12 days prior to menstrual bleeding and/or the absence of corpus luteum determined through ultrasonography, for three consecutive cycles. Ovulation is confirmed when serum progesterone measurements are greater than 5 ng/ml [10 nmol/l]. However, inappropriate timing of progesterone measurements will obviously lead to an inaccurate diagnosis of anovulation, progesterone measurement not being, in any case, the common practice.

In a significant percentage of studies, women who reported less than ten menstrual cycles per year were considered as anovulatory. The limitation of this commonly used approach is that it yields a large number of false positive and false negative results in PCOS study groups. False negatives are considered to be those women with more than 10 cycles per year, but who could be anovulatory, especially in the case of frequent menstruation; false positive women include those with 8 cycles, but all ovulatory. Furthermore, ovulatory dysfunction may be present in women with PCOS who report regular menstrual cycles. Accordingly, menstrual history alone is insufficient for definition of PCOS phenotypes in women whose cycles are regular, especially in the presence of hyperandrogenism. In the event of doubt, progesterone evaluation should be carried out.

It should also be borne in mind that in a normally ovulating woman, the loss of one to two ovulations per year is considered a natural phenomenon. Moreover, central obesity and insulin resistance are strongly associated with anovulation and a transition between anovulation and ovulation has been documented in women with PCOS undergoing caloric reduction programs leading to relatively rapid weight loss. It is hence possible that a woman considered to be anovulatory may ovulate after a 5–10% loss of BMI, this being a situation that the clinician should always take into consideration for both diagnostic and therapeutic reasons [11].

Polycystic Ovarian Morphology

As shown in table 1, confirmation of the existence of polycystic ovaries requires either the visualization of 12 or more follicles measuring 2–9 mm or ovarian volume bigger than 10 cm^3. Both situations are suggestive of PCOM even if they are detected in the one ovary. This definition is more useful than the previous one, whereby the assessment of stromal echogenicity and/or follicle distribution pattern were necessary characteristics that have been abandoned due to their high degree of subjectivity.

However, ovarian volume and, in particular, follicle measurement is a subjective process highly dependent on the accuracy, experience, and attentiveness of the ultrasonographer. In an interesting study conducted by Amer's group, it was found that an agreement for PCOM between observers was found in only 50% of cases. It must be underlined that the cutoff value of 12 follicles was found to have increased specificity (99%) and sensitivity (75%) for PCOM in only one study. Other studies have not reproduced these findings, increasing the noise of ultrasonography use in PCOS diagnosis. For example, in a large study of more than 600 women with PCOS and 100 controls, 12 follicles per ovary were found in about half of controls. As a consequence, among gynecologists PCOM is a very strong factor for PCOS diagnosis, whereas according to endocrinologists it constitutes a supportive but not a definitive tool for diagnosis. Furthermore, several reproductive endocrinologists suggest different criteria in clinical practice, such as >20 follicles per ovary or increased stroma/total area ratio, whereas medical imaging specialists use older criteria (stroma/follicles pattern) because of their long familiarization with them.

Furthermore, since follicles number and ovarian volume are highly correlated with the current use of oral contraceptives (OCPs), an interval of 3 months after OCP discontinuation is the minimum time needed before ovarian ultrasonography is carried out. Similar actions in ovarian morphology should be expected in the case of metformin administration and, to a lesser degree, with antiandrogen treatment.

Another factor that affects ovarian morphology is age. About 20% of women of reproductive age display PCOM without any other sign of PCOS (hyperandrogenism and anovulation), this fraction being still higher in adolescents among whom 40–50% of girls display PCOM, which, however, resolves through years. Finally, we should keep in mind that a spontaneous ovulation is sufficient to totally correct ovarian morphology, especially follicle number. In order to ensure the best quality of ultrasound in

PCOS, some useful guidelines were published in 2003: (a) the use of state-of-the-art equipment is required and must be operated by trained personnel; (b) if possible, the transvaginal approach is to be preferred, particularly in obese patients; (c) in regularly menstruating women, ultrasound should be scanned in the early follicular phase (days 3–5), and in oligo /amenorrheic women, either at random or between days 3–5 after progestogen-induced bleeding; (d) in the event that a dominant follicle (>10 mm) or a corpus luteum are detected, the scan should be repeated during the next cycle, and (e) follicle number should be estimated both in longitudinal, transverse, and anteroposterior cross-sections of the ovaries. Follicle size should be expressed as the mean of the diameters measured in the three sections.

In conclusion, ovarian morphology, although mandatory for PCOS diagnosis and further consolidated with the Rotterdam criteria, requires a careful approach. An experienced and meticulous ultrasonographer thoroughly familiar with current criteria is a prerequisite. For optimal results, a detailed report recording the number of follicles and ovarian volume should always be demanded, while medical terms that are now outdated, such as increased stroma, micropolycystic ovaries, etc. should be avoided. Finally, knowledge of age and current drug use is absolutely essential for ultrasound evaluation [12, 13].

Cardiovascular Risk, Metabolic and Hormonal Profile Comparison of Four Phenotypes of PCOS Based on the Rotterdam Criteria

The introduction of the new PCOS phenotypes according to the Rotterdam criteria was accompanied by considerable apprehension as regards PCOS long-term sequelae. As has been clearly shown, already as from the 1990s women with PCOS diagnosed according to the NIH criteria exhibited an unfavorable metabolic/hormonal milieu associated with a cluster of several CV risk factors such as oxidative stress, dyslipidemia, subclinical inflammation, and impaired fibrinolysis. Furthermore, Shaw and colleagues recently reported that postmenopausal women with classic PCOS (hyperandrogenism and chronic anovulation) display a higher rate of CV morbidity and mortality. A fascinating finding of this study was the observation that higher CV morbidity/mortality was not observed in women with a history of isolated either hyperandrogenemia or menstrual irregularities. Hence, only classic PCOS seems to be associated with increased CV risk. This study highlighted the need for lifetime follow-up of these patients and stressed the need for early identification of these factors and therapeutic modalities aiming to reduce CV risk.

However, it has not as yet been elucidated in women with PCOM, which are the metabolic implications, and if CV risk in phenotype C ('ovulatory' PCOS) or phenotype D ('mild' PCOS) is comparable to those diagnosed with NIH criteria. The design of prospective follow-up studies from adolescence to menopause of women with different PCOS phenotypes will provide a definitive answer to this issue. It must be underlined that this issue is of utmost importance given that, with the use of the new criteria and also depending on the population recruited, 20–25% of women carrying PCOS diagnosis may have ovulatory PCOS (C), or a percentage ranging from 10 to 20% may suffer from non-hyperandrogenic PCOS (D).

Regarding hormonal milieu, most studies suggest that LH levels and LH-to-FSH ratio are higher in normal-weight and overweight women with classic PCOS phenotypes than women with similar BMI but the newer phenotypes. Panidis' group suggested that the higher LH concentrations have been attributed to the higher androgen levels, which desensitize the hypothalamus to the negative feedback regulation by progesterone [14]. Androgen concentrations (testosterone, androstenedione, dehydroepiandrosterone) have been found to be lower in phenotype D than in the other three phenotypes, but higher than normal in ovulating, non-hyperandrogenic women. A detailed study by Legro's group examined the impact of both features of PCOM (ovarian volume and follicles number) on metabolic/hormonal parameters. Although they noted that follicle number is a better discriminator of ovarian volume between PCOS and control women, they concluded that neither morphology nor ovarian volume was associated with distinctive metabolic phenotypes. On the other hand, Laven's group explored the impact of oligo-anovulation or anovulation on ovarian dysfunction. They found elevated levels of testosterone, free androgen index, and total follicle count in anovulatory patients as well as a better response to clomiphene treatment. They consequently concluded that ovulatory women with PCOS exhibit a milder phenotype compared with anovulatory PCOS patients. This point is of major clinical importance since the issue of anovulation should not be neglected, while in the case of a patient with phenotype D, the clinician should be aware of possible reproductive dysfunction [15].

With respect to metabolic profile and CV risk factors, several studies suggested that women with PCOS based on the NIH criteria exhibit a detrimental profile compared to newer phenotypes. Usually, women with classic PCOS are heavier, but when comparisons of groups were made between groups matched for age and BMI, it was obvious that the degree of dyslipidemia, central adiposity, insulin resistance, and metabolic syndrome prevalence was significantly higher in women with classic PCOS phenotype. However, the prevalence of metabolic syndrome and degree of insulin resistance in phenotype D, although elevated, is closer to control subjects than to the other three phenotypes. Available data suggest that oligoanovulatory patients with polycystic ovaries but without hyperandogenemia (phenotype D) display mild endocrine abnormalities, but not the metabolic features of PCOS. Specifically, women with this phenotype usually display normal insulin sensitivity and a metabolic profile similar to age- and BMI-matched normal women [16, 17].

On the other hand, as regards phenotype C, a recent study from Turkey evaluating not only CV risk factors but also carotid intima-media thickness reported that in women with polycystic ovaries and hyperandrogenemia CV risk was lower than in other phenotypes [18]. In agreement with the above are data originating from

Amato et al. [19] who, through the evaluation of the visceral adiposity index (VAI), found that oligomenorrhea was associated with increased CV risk. VAI is a mathematical model of CV risk estimation determined by using BMI, waist circumference, triglycerides, and HDL cholesterol parameters. This marker of visceral adipose dysfunction showed a strong association with both the rate of peripheral glucose utilization and visceral adipose tissue and has a strong independent association with CV events. These findings are in disagreement with the general belief that phenotypes with androgen excess have the highest CV risk. However, one may hypothesize that the above controversial data arise due to the nature of PCOS, and women with hyperandrogenemia and PCOM may develop through time anovulation, especially if they gain some weight. This logical approach underlines the gap of understanding regarding the nature of the syndrome based on available data. It is not known if women with phenotypes C or D develop frank PCOS (NIH criteria) later in their life or what is the actual CV risk of women with these phenotypes.

A Critical Reappraisal of PCOS Definition and Phenotypes – Impact on Cardiovascular Risk

There is accumulating evidence that PCOS constitutes a continuum spectrum starting from the early prepubertal years and continuing after menopause. Specifically, girls with a history of premature pubarche exhibit metabolic and hormonal derangements usually encountered in PCOS and are at increased risk of developing PCOS after puberty compared to their normal peers. Furthermore, women with a history of PCOS display a significantly higher rate of CV events after menopause, suggesting that the increased CV risk observed during the reproductive years is actually transformed into clinical events.

PCOS diagnosis peaks through the second and third decade of life, since the vast majority of patients seek medical help mainly due to clinical signs of hyperandrogenism and/or oligomenorrhea. If the diagnosis is based strictly on the NIH criteria, a prevalence of 6–8% of women of reproductive age will be diagnosed with PCOS, while this number will rise to 15–25% with the use of the Rotterdam criteria. The fact that the cost of evaluating this large number of patients is high but the long-term benefit of ameliorating the hormonal and metabolic profile in quality of life and of reducing CV risk is significant remains a challenge for the clinician.

However, the major problem with PCOS definition based on the Rotterdam criteria is the defining of the different phenotypes and their impact on mortality and related morbidities. We at present lack some essential information that would enable us to judge the utility of the Rotterdam criteria: namely, do women with Rotterdam PCOS transfer from the one phenotype to another, and specifically from ovulatory PCOS to anovulatory PCOS, and how does this transition affect their health status in the long term? If the answer to the above query is affirmative, then

it can be postulated that women who have presented once with a mild phenotype may at a later stage of their life develop a worse and severe phenotype, with the known adverse sequelae. Although core data answering these questions are thus far not available, it is hypothesized from the pathophysiological point of view that women transfer from the one phenotype to another depending on their exposure to several factors, such as increment of bodyweight, dietary intake, and exercise habits.

It has been clearly reported by a large number of different research groups that anovulatory PCOS display a notably worse metabolic and hormonal profile compared to ovulating PCOS, but we are not aware how common this is and if predicting factors exist among phenotypes. One may argue that the presence of polycystic ovary in ultrasound may be a sign of inherent ovarian dysregulation and that these women have 'intrinsic' PCOS diagnosed as from menarche due to anovulation, whereas in other women external factors and, most commonly, weight gain yield an apparent PCOS diagnosis. However, in a recent study conducted by our group, we investigated the impact of emergence of menstrual irregularities on metabolic and hormonal derangements observed in PCOS. Specifically, in half of them oligomenorrhea was observed starting from menarche, while in the other half it presented at least 3 years after menarche. When these women were evaluated at 25 years of age, it was found that both metabolic and hormonal profile were comparable among them, independently of the timing of menstrual irregularities commencement. This study shows that the cardinal hormonal/metabolic PCOS manifestations associated with the increased CV risk of the syndrome are similar at a later period of time, despite the time of diagnosis [20]. However, it is not known yet if women with different PCOS phenotypes based on the Rotterdam criteria are exposed to the same degree of CV risk. If so, then the use of ultrasound, despite the abovementioned limitations, will probably help to identify these women early and to reduce CV risk by appropriate lifestyle modifications. Therefore, an intense follow-up may prove to be beneficial also in patients with the new PCOS phenotypes. Lifestyle modifications, such as restriction of caloric intake and exercise, should be encouraged with the aim of reducing long-term CV risk.

Differential Diagnosis of PCOS

As it has been stated, PCOS is a syndrome and a diagnosis of exclusion. Accordingly, although common, it cannot be diagnosed before the exclusion of other endocrinopathies, such as NC-CAH, Cushing syndrome, acromegaly, hyperprolactinemia, hypothyroidism, premature ovarian failure, virilizing adrenal or ovarian tumor, and a drug-related condition. This workup, although both expensive and time-consuming, is mandatory in most cases. In this paragraph, a critical approach to PCOS diagnosis and recommendations as to differential diagnosis will be provided.

Diagnosis of PCOS is guided on a clinical basis through personal history. Since PCOS clinical findings represent a continuum of symptoms, the occurrence of a gradual development of signs of hyperandrogenism accompanied by slight deterioration of menstrual cycle, especially in the case of weight gain, are highly suggestive of PCOS. Furthermore, a family history of hyperandrogenism, oligomenorrhea, and diabetes mellitus type 2 are found with increased prevalence in subjects with PCOS, and should be taken into consideration. In cases of women with a history of intrauterine growth retardation and/or premature pubarche (appearance of pubic hair prior to age 8), particular vigilance is needed. These girls are at increased risk of developing PCOS during adolescence and a thorough evaluation to exclude NC-CAH is required [21].

The most critical issue in the differential diagnosis of other hyperandrogenic disorders is the patient's history. A rapid deterioration of menstruation accompanied by signs of accelerating virilization with abrupt worsening are indicative of an androgen-producing neoplasm. In this case, testosterone and DHEAS values will lead the diagnosis. Regarding exclusion of thyroid dysfunction, any alteration of the menstrual cycle towards oligo- or amenorrhea, as well as the presentation of the classic findings of hyper- and hypothyroidism, will be suggestive. The combination of TSH and thyroxine values possesses great sensitivity for unraveling both causes of dysthyroidism, and is considered basic in the differential diagnosis of PCOS.

Hyperprolactinemia represents a trickier situation, given that 20–40% of PCOS patients display slightly elevated prolactin levels. This 2-fold rise is a result of positive feedback of unopposed estrogen action in the pituitary and may sometimes be accompanied by breast tenderness, bloating, and mastodynia. Usually, no further investigations are needed, since menstruation control with either OCPs or metformin will normalize prolactin levels. However, in the case of headaches, visual problems, and constant elevation of prolactin levels, an MRI should be carried out in order to exclude pituitary adenoma or pituitary stalk interruption due to other causes. Additionally, the clinician should be aware of the 'hook' phenomenon which leads to upper normal prolactin values in patients with macroprolactinomas, this due to kit antibodies consumption.

Adrenal dysfunction may be presented as PCOS in either Cushing syndrome or NC-CAH. Cushing syndrome is rare, but the classic symptoms of central obesity and striae will not guide the diagnosis, since they occur later in the course of disease than menstrual irregularities and hyperandrogenemia. In the event that clinical suspicion of Cushing is strong, based on abrupt menses deterioration, edema, erythema, etc., the overnight dexamethasone test is a very accurate screening test, while 24-hour urine cortisol levels will confirm the diagnosis.

However, the most complicated pathologic entity of PCOS diagnosis is the exclusion of NC-CAH. In several studies, women of reproductive age with NC-CAH display a PCOS-like syndrome, namely hyperandrogenemia, ovulatory dysfunction,

infertility, and PCOM in ultrasound. The link between PCOS and NC-CAH has not as yet been clarified, though it has been tentatively attributed to excess adrenal androgens which disrupt gonadotropin release and modify ovarian steroid synthesis. Moreover, a direct effect of adrenal steroids on the ovary leading to anovulation and overproduction of ovarian androgens has also been proposed. Data on the frequency of NC-CAH or *CYP21A2* heterozygosity, based on molecular studies in a large number of women with PCOS, although limited, show that about <5% of women presenting with polycystic ovary-like syndrome carry 21-hydroxylase gene mutations.

Azziz and Zacur suggested that basal values of 17OHP lower than 2 ng/ml (6.1 nmol/l) should rule out NC-CAH, and this concentration is generally accepted as the upper normal value. However, in the study by Bachega's group, out of 58 subjects suspected of having NC-CAH based on basal and stimulated levels of 17OHP higher than 1.6 and 10 ng/ml (4.8 and 30 nmol/l), respectively, the diagnosis was confirmed by molecular studies in only 36. Additionally, Bidet and colleagues reported that in a large cohort of women with NC-CAH, 8% displayed basal 17OHP values lower than 2 ng/ml (6.1 nmol/l). Hence, it should be considered that false results can be obtained with the basal currently applied hormonal criteria for the diagnosis of NC-CAH.

For that reason, the use of the Synacthen test is very helpful for NC-CAH exclusion. Bachega's group suggested that the lowest peak of 17-OHP after ACTH in fully genotyped subjects was 17 ng/ml (51.5 nmol/l), while Azziz et al. [1] reported that the level of 10 ng/ml [30 nmol/l] is the lower threshold in patients with NC-CAH. The latter value is in accordance with data obtained from the study of Escobar-Morreale, and Bidet's groups, derived from cohorts of hyperandrogenic women. 17OH progesterone values after ACTH stimulation is a prerequisite for NC-CAH, especially in women with PCOS with a history of premature pubarche. Furthermore, when NC-CAH diagnosis is completed, molecular evaluation is obligatory for prenatal advice and appropriate management through gestation.

Diagnosing PCOS in Adolescence

The diagnosis of the syndrome in adolescence demands a high degree of circumspection and clinical experience to overcome diagnostic difficulties especially encountered in this population. One major problem is the menstrual irregularities observed in adolescents. In healthy adolescents, half of the cycles are anovulatory in the first year after menarche, but tends to normalize through time. Although there is the general belief that oligomenorrhea and anovulatory cycles are to be expected in adolescence, it is noteworthy that if menstrual irregularities persist 2 years after menarche, then the risk for PCOS is extremely high (70% of cases). Despite menstrual cyclicity, an adolescent's common complaint is dysfunctional uterine bleeding, clinically

expressed as menstrual flow greater than 80 ml per cycle or subjectively the use of more than 6 full pads or tampons per day. This situation should not be confused with PCOS, and the combination of ultrasound with androgen evaluation will differentiate this diagnosis.

With regard to hyperandrogenemia and signs of hyperandrogenism, there exist some specific age-related limitations. In the vast majority of adolescents, slight acne and hirsutism lasting a period of 1–2 years, which is anticipated and probably reflects transient functional hyperandrogenism of adolescence, is not of significant clinical importance. Despite the above-described difficulties in assessing biochemical hyperandrogenism, there is a lack of normative data for the adolescent population. This parameter is of great importance, given that during adolescence an increased frequency of Gn-RH pulse generator is observed, leading to higher LH pulse amplitude, which is connected with higher androgen production. Furthermore, during the peripubertal period fat accumulation accompanied by higher leptin levels is observed, this being a prerequisite for the initiation of the reproductive axis. However, as is known, increased adiposity aggravates hyperinsulinemia and consequently affects positively circulating androgen levels through the amplification of ovarian theca cell androgen production and the decrease in SHBG levels [22].

Finally, signs of insulin resistance should be noted. The presence of acanthosis nigricans, velvety and pigmented areas of the skin, especially in the axilla and at the nape of the neck, indicates insulin resistance. However, it must also be borne in mind that ethnic differences have been reported between different populations so that presentation of acanthosis nigricans with the same degree of insulinemia is highly dependent on ethnicity.

These complaints and clinical findings should be carefully evaluated and an ultrasound will help the diagnosis. However, there are some limitations regarding the use of ultrasound in adolescence. First of all, during puberty polycystic ovaries should be distinguished from multicystic ovaries, which occur normally. In the latter, a larger size of cysts and thick ovarian stroma is expected. Furthermore, the use of the abdominal instead of transvaginal route in teenage virgins decreases ultrasound sensitivity.

Towards a Tailor-Made Approach to Different PCOS Phenotypes

The different phenotypic expression of PCOS requires a tailor-made approach and management. It is obvious that in the case of anovulation combined with hyperandrogenism, the management will be directed in accordance with the specific needs of the patient. In the event of infertility, metformin initiation and clomiphene administration significantly increase the possibility of pregnancy. On the other hand, if oligomenorrhea is the dominant syndrome, metformin has the ability to improve ovulation in 60–70% of patients. In the event that hyperandrogenic signs have prompted the request for medical assistance, oral contraceptives with or without antiandrogen prescription comprise the usual approach.

However, these classic therapeutic modalities are today disputed under the prism of the newer phenotypes. In the case of ovulatory PCOS, hyperandrogenism per se does not necessitate treatment for many patients since they tolerate this situation well. Furthermore, in many patients with oligoanovulation and polycystic ovarian morphology, the diagnosis is usually made spontaneously during regular gynecologic exams. In these two phenotypes, the woman does not consider herself as a patient, especially if a positive family history of either hyperandrogenism or oligomenorrhea exists. As mentioned above, the cardiometabolic risk in newer phenotypes has not been well defined. However, we should keep in mind that in PCOS a continuum of symptoms and abnormalities is displayed starting with hyperandrogenism and anovulation in the second and the third decade of life, which are transformed to metabolic disease (dyslipidemia, hyperglycemia) later on. Furthermore, long-term follow-up of women with PCOS (NIH criteria) revealed that a significant percentage (40%) would develop impaired glucose tolerance or type 2 diabetes during the fourth decade of life. The risk for diabetes in PCOS is 10 times higher than in their age- and BMI-matched peers and reflects the metabolic abnormalities encountered in this population [23]. Since in newer phenotypes it is not known yet if they will subsequently develop the full spectrum of PCOS based on NIH criteria and the available data do not exclude the possibility of increased cardiometabolic risk, the clinician should provide appropriate guidance to patients. Exercise is today recognized worldwide as being the cornerstone of decreasing insulin resistance and the occurrence of diabetes and CV incidents. Furthermore, in the case of treatment modalities including oral contraceptives and antiandrogens, their use should be time-limited, and they should be administered for a specific reason since the vast majority of these agents will display well-known atherogenic properties. By contrast, metformin has proven sufficient to reduce long-term risk of diabetes development, and its use has shown beneficial effects in lowering CV markers, not only in adolescents and adult women with PCOS but also in prepubertal girls with premature pubarche. However, the clinician should be aware of metformin role in reducing B_{12} levels, and periodic examination is warranted.

Impact of Nutrition on PCOS Phenotypes and Metabolic/Hormonal Abnormalities – A Potential Role for Advanced Glycated End Products

Regarding the nutritional approach, healthy dietary habits should be encouraged. A balanced, healthy nutritional program based on the Mediterranean diet together with regular exercise has been shown to considerably ameliorate cardiometabolic risk in both PCOS and normal ovulating, though not in hyperandrogenemic women

[23, 24]. Meanwhile, advanced glycated end products (AGEs) have been recognized as potent endocrine disruptors. Endocrine disruptor designates any molecule found in an environment, which may interfere with hormone biosynthesis, metabolism, or action, resulting in a deviation from normal homeostasis and/or reproduction. AGEs fulfill these principles since they exhibit strong oxidative, proinflammatory, and proatherogenic properties and have been associated with increased CV morbidity in both diabetic and nondiabetic subjects. Dietary intake of AGEs is high, particularly in the West, given that they are found in large quantities in heat-treated foods that are abundant in Western diets.

With regard to PCOS patients, AGEs have been found to be elevated in comparison to those in normal women [25]. Additionally, in women with classic phenotype, serum AGE levels are higher than in their counterparts with the newer ovulating phenotype, despite the fact that age, BMI, and degree of insulin resistance was comparable between these groups. On the other hand, in those with anovulation and polycystic ovarian morphology, AGE levels were similar to controls.

Furthermore, AGEs appear to have a differential role between PCOS anovulatory versus ovulatory phenotypes: not only are their serum levels higher but they also follow the same pattern as anti-müllerian hormone (a specific marker of ovulatory dysfunction in PCOS) [26]. On clinical grounds, these observations are in accordance with recent study findings in which high AGE levels in follicular fluid and serum are correlated negatively with fertility rate. These findings suggest interference of AGEs in the ovulatory process as well as their differential role between PCOS phenotypes.

Conclusions

PCOS is a lifelong disease. It is presented with a continuum spectrum of symptoms and is connected with significant cardiometabolic risk. However, following the introduction of the Rotterdam criteria, more phenotypes have been disclosed for which the exact impact on mortality, associated morbidities, and quality of life has not as yet been elucidated. Given that we do not know if a woman presenting with polycystic ovaries on ultrasound and hyperandrogenism or anovulation will develop at a later stage of her life the full-blown syndrome, great care should be taken in her evaluation. In the interest of implementing a tailor-made diagnostic approach, the clinician is recommended to take a meticulous, in-depth medical history accompanied by a detailed clinical examination, all of which will reduce the need for an expensive and laborious workup. Most importantly, the clinician needs not only to address the problem which prompted the woman to seek medical assistance but should also strongly recommend women with PCOS to embrace a healthful lifestyle involving adoption of healthy nutritional habits and regular exercise.

References

1 Azziz R CF, Dewailly D, Diamanti-Kandarakis E, Escobar-Morreale HF, Futterweit W, Janssen OE, Legro RS, Norman RJ, Taylor AE, Witchel SF: Task Force on the Phenotype of the Polycystic Ovary Syndrome of the Androgen Excess and PCOS Society. The Androgen Excess and PCOS Society criteria for the polycystic ovary syndrome: the complete task force report. Fertil Steril 2009;91:456.

2 Rotterdam ESHRE/ASRM-Sponsored PCOS Consensus Workshop Group. Revised 2003 consensus on diagnostic criteria and long-term health risks related to polycystic ovary syndrome (PCOS). Hum Reprod 2004;19:41.

3 Cussons AJ, Bronwyn GA, Stuckey G, Walsh JP, Burke V, Norman RJ: Polycystic ovarian syndrome: marked differences between endocrinologists and gynecologists in diagnosis and management. Clin Endocrinol 2005;62:289.

4 Diamanti-Kandarakis E, Kouli CR, Bergiele AT, Filandra FA, Tsianateli TC, Spina GG, Zapanti ED, Bartzis MI: A survey of the polycystic ovary syndrome in the Greek island of Lesbos: hormonal and metabolic profile. J Clin Endocrinol Metab 1999; 84:4006.

5 Broekmans FJ, Knauff EA, Valkenburg O, Laven JS, Eijkemans MJ, Fauser BC: PCOS according to the Rotterdam consensus criteria: change in prevalence among WHO-II anovulation and association with metabolic factors. Br J Obstet Gynecol 2006;113: 1210.

6 Ibanez L, de Zegher F, Potau N: Anovulation after precocious pubarche: early markers and time course in adolescence. J Clin Endocrinol Metab 1999;84: 2691.

7 Shaw LJ, Bairey Merz CN, Azziz R, Stanczyk FZ, Sopko G, Braunstein GD, Kelsey SF, Kip KE, Cooper-Dehoff RM, Johnson BD, et al: Postmenopausal women with a history of irregular menses and elevated androgen measurements at high risk for worsening cardiovascular event-free survival: results from the National Institutes of Health – National Heart, Lung, and Blood Institute sponsored Women's Ischemia Syndrome Evaluation. J Clin Endocrinol Metab 2008;93:1276.

8 Vermeulen A, Verdonck L, Kaufman JM: A critical evaluation of simple methods for the estimation of free testosterone in serum. J Clin Endocrinol Metab 1999;84:3666.

9 Livadas S, Boutzios G, Economou F, Alexandraki K, Xyrafis X, Christou M, Zerva A, Karachalios A, Tantalaki E, Diamanti-Kandarakis E: The effect of oral micronized progesterone on hormonal and metabolic parameters in anovulatory patients with polycystic ovary syndrome. Fertil Steril 2010; 94:242.

10 Yildiz BO, Bolour S, Woods A, Moore A, Azziz R: Visually scoring hirsutism. Hum Repr Update 2010; 16:51.

11 Malcolm CE, Cumming DC: Does anovulation exist in eumenorrheic women? Obstet Gynecol 2003; 102:317.

12 Jonard S, Robert Y, Cortet-Rudelli C, Pigny P, Decanter C, Dewailly D: Ultrasound examination of polycystic ovaries: is it worth counting the follicles? Hum Reprod 2003;18:598.

13 Balen AH, Laven JS, Tan SL, Dewailly D: Ultrasound assessment of the polycystic ovary: international consensus definitions. Hum Reprod Update 2003; 9:505–514.

14 Katsikis I, Karkanaki A, Misichronis G, Delkos D, Kandaraki EA, Panidis D: Phenotypic expression, body mass index and insulin resistance in relation to LH levels in women with polycystic ovary syndrome. Eur J Obstet Gynecol Reprod Biol 2011; 156:181.

15 Burgers JA, Fong SL, Louwers YV, Valkenburg O, de Jong FH, Fauser JM, Laven JS: Oligoovulatory and anovulatory cycles in women with polycystic ovary syndrome (PCOS): what's the difference? Clin Endocrinol Metab 2010;95:E485.

16 Diamanti-Kandarakis E, Panidis D: Unravelling the phenotypic map of polycystic ovary syndrome (PCOS): a prospective study of 634 women with PCOS. Clin Endocrinol (Oxf) 2007;67:735.

17 Moran L, Teede H: Metabolic features of the reproductive phenotypes of polycystic ovary syndrome. Hum Reprod Update 2009;15:477.

18 Dilbaz B, Ozkaya E, Cinar M, Cakir E, Dilbaz S: Cardiovascular disease risk characteristics of the main polycystic ovary syndrome phenotypes. Endocrine 2011;39:272.

19 Amato MC, Verghi M, Galluzzo A, Giordano C: The oligomenorrhoic phenotypes of polycystic ovary syndrome are characterized by a high visceral adiposity index: a likely condition of cardiometabolic risk. Hum Reprod 2011;26:1486.

20 Livadas S, Christou M, Economou F, Karachalios A, Xyrafis X, Boutzios G, Zerva A, Tantalaki E, Palimeri S, Diamanti-Kandarakis E: Menstrual irregularities in PCOS. Does it matter when it starts? Exp Clin Endocrinol Diabetes 2011;119:334.

21 Diamanti-Kandarakis E: Polycystic ovarian syndrome: pathophysiology, molecular aspects and clinical implications. Expert Rev Mol Med 2008; 10:e3.

22 Diamanti-Kandarakis E, Christakou C, Palioura E, Kandaraki E, Livadas S: Does polycystic ovary syndrome start in childhood? Pediatr Endocrinol Rev 2008;5:904.

23 Legro RS, Kunselman AR, Dodson WC, Dunaif A: Prevalence and predictors of risk for type 2 diabetes mellitus and impaired glucose tolerance in polycystic ovary syndrome: a prospective, controlled study in 254 affected women. J Clin Endocrinol Metab 1999;84:165.
24 Norman RJ, Davies MJ, Lord J, Moran LJ: The role of lifestyle modification in polycystic ovary syndrome. Trends Endocrinol Metab 2002;13:251.
25 Diamanti-Kandarakis E, Katsikis I, Piperi C, Kandaraki E, Piouka A, Papavassiliou AG, Panidis D: Increased serum advanced glycation end-products is a distinct finding in lean women with polycystic ovary syndrome (PCOS). Clin Endocrinol (Oxf) 2008b;69:634–641.
26 Diamanti-Kandarakis E, Piouka A, Livadas S, Piperi C, Katsikis I, Papavassiliou AG, Panidis D: Anti-Mullerian hormone is associated with advanced glycosylated end products in lean women with polycystic ovary syndrome. Eur J Endocrinol 2009;160:847.

Evanthia Diamanti-Kandarakis, MD, PhD
Endocrine Unit, Third Department of Internal Medicine, Medical School
National and Kapodistrian University of Athens
1A Zefyrou Street Ekali
GR–14578 Athens (Greece)
Tel. +30 210 6778333, E-Mail e.diamanti.kandarakis@gmail.com

Macut D, Pfeifer M, Yildiz BO, Diamanti-Kandarakis E (eds): Polycystic Ovary Syndrome. Novel Insights into Causes and Therapy. Front Horm Res. Basel, Karger, 2013, vol 40, pp 22–27

Pathophysiology of Polycystic Ovary Syndrome: The Role of Hyperandrogenism

Sophie Catteau-Jonard · Didier Dewailly

Service de Gynécologie Endocrinienne et Médecine de la Reproduction, Hôpital Jeanne de Flandre, CHU de Lille, Lille, France

Abstract

The cardinal features of polycystic ovary syndrome (PCOS) are hyperandrogenism and oligoanovulation. The increase in ovarian androgen production is a fundamental characteristic of PCOS and, although enigmatic, it is at the heart of one of the major issues about the pathophysiology of PCOS, i.e. whether it has developmental origins or not. Intraovarian androgens are designated as primarily responsible for the follicle excess. The defective selection of a dominant follicle in anovulatory patients results from both an insufficient secretion of FSH and a local inhibition of FSH action. Anti-müllerian hormone (AMH) seems to be involved in the latter by repressing the FSH-dependent aromatase activity. AMH level is increased in PCOS because of the follicle excess and increased production per follicle. Therefore, in anovulatory patients, serum FSH, although at low to normal plasma concentrations, would not be able to induce a decrease in AMH sufficient to allow the expression of aromatase. In conclusion, the fundamental anomaly of PCOS is still unknown, but it can be hypothesized that any genetic, epigenetic or environmental factor leading to intraovarian hyperandrogenism can result in PCOS.

Polycystic ovary syndrome (PCOS) is the most common cause of anovulation, infertility and hyperandrogenism in women. Indeed, 5–10% of women of reproductive age are affected [1]. Despite considerable efforts to determine the cause, the pathophysiology of PCOS remains poorly understood, but evidence is accumulating to suggest that central abnormalities of PCOS are primarily ovarian [1]. Knowledge of the mechanisms leading to PCOS is one of the major issues of Clinical Research in Endocrine Gynecology and Reproductive Medicine.

The cardinal features of PCOS are hyperandrogenism and oligoanovulation. The hyperandrogenism is becoming more like the 'heart' of PCOS, and the first impact would be impaired folliculogenesis. Hyperinsulinism secondary to insulin resistance [see the chapter about obesity and metabolic syndrome by Carmina, pp. 40–50] is not part of the syndrome. It is not a causal factor, but rather a '2nd hit' neither necessary nor sufficient for the formation of a PCOS, except in cases of extreme hyperinsulinemia.

Hyperandrogenism

The increase in ovarian androgen production is a fundamental characteristic of PCOS [2]. It lays on an excessive theca cell activity, whose explanation is less and less involving extraovarian factors and more and more intraovarian factors.

The elevation of serum LH is a classic but inconsistent feature of PCOS. It is the result of both the acceleration of the frequency of LH pulses and the increase of the amplitude of these pulses [3]. It is less and less regarded as a primary phenomenon. Recent data suggest that it results from a lack of negative feedback of estradiol or progesterone. This lack of feedback could be due to the action of androgen excess on the hypothalamic-pituitary axis in the peripubertal period [4]. Excess androgens may reduce the sensitivity of the GnRH pulse generator to sex steroid inhibition in susceptible individuals, resulting in increased GnRH pulse frequency and subsequent abnormalities in gonadotropin secretion, ovarian androgen production, and ovulatory function. Hyperinsulinemia may also be considered as a non-ovarian factor of hyperandrogenism by amplifying the effects of LH on steroid production by theca interstitial cells [5]. In vitro, insulin directly stimulates ovarian androgen secretion via its effects on the cytochrome P450 C17-α. In vivo, insulin-sensitizing agent or weight loss lowers plasma androgen levels through the decrease in insulin concentrations [5]. On the other hand, the IGF system does not seem to have an important role in ovarian hyperandrogenism [6].

Among the putative intraovarian factors, the inhibins may also be involved in intraovarian hyperandrogenism of polycystic ovaries (PCO) via a paracrine effect through which granulosa cells (GC) modulate the synthesis of androgens by the theca interstitial cells [7]. However, no recent study has addressed this issue.

In fact, long-term cultures suggest that the transcription of genes encoding steroidogenic enzymes are naturally 'upregulated' specifically in the theca cells of PCO, but none of the enzymatic steps is affected [8]. This leads to an increased production of androgens and progestins. Therefore, although the hyperandrogenism of PCOS is subject to a phenomenon of familial aggregation, with a mode of transmission that appears to be autosomal dominant, this 'up-regulation' is unlikely due to the anomaly of a single gene encoding a precise steroidogenic enzyme. The recent progress in the genetics of PCOS, using the GWAS approach, focuses on susceptibility loci that do not seem to imply genes involved in androgen synthesis, metabolism or sensitivity [see the chapter about genetics of PCOS by Barber and Franks, pp. 28–39].

Although its mechanism is still enigmatic, the primary ovarian hyperandrogenism is at the heart of one of the major recent issues about the pathophysiology of PCOS, i.e. whether it has developmental origins or not [9]. This theory originates from animal studies showing that after fetal exposition to high doses of androgens, an endocrine and metabolic phenotype develops at puberty, resembling human PCOS [reviewed in 9]. This theory implies that under some genetic and/or epigenetic influence(s), the human fetal ovary would be able to masculinize some organs such as the hypothalamus and the pancreas and even itself, disrupting folliculogenesis (see below). This would program the individual for developing an endocrine and metabolic phenotype of PCOS at puberty [reviewed in 9].

The Disordered Folliculogenesis

The observation by Hughesdon [10] of a number of growing follicles up to the stage 2–5 mm two to three times more in PCO than in normal ovaries is certainly an old one, but still essential. It has been confirmed more recently in cortical biopsies [11].

This anomaly is associated with a second phenomenon that is the growth arrest of these follicles when they reach the stage 4–7 mm. This suggests that there are essentially two anomalies affecting folliculogenesis in PCO [12]: excessive follicular growth on the one hand, and on the other hand, inhibition within the excessive cohort of the emergence of a dominant follicle. The second anomaly is called 'follicular arrest'.

Excessive Early Follicular Growth

Knowing their importance in the growth of small follicles, intraovarian androgens are designated as primarily responsible for this phenomenon of follicle excess. Experimental studies in rhesus female monkeys receiving high doses of testosterone or dihydrotestosterone suggest that androgens promote the growth of small follicles in the primate ovary and reduce GC apoptosis [13]. This may be related to some clinical observations. The congenital adrenal hyperplasia, virilizing tumors and the administration of exogenous androgens (in trans-sexual female to male) are associated with a greater number of antral follicles, the same as those observed in PCO [14].

Finally, the ultrasound data in our patients with PCOS [15], indicating a positive correlation between the number of 2- to 5-mm follicles and serum testosterone and androstenedione levels, reinforce the hypothesis that the increase in small follicles is due to the trophic effect of androgens, either increased locally in the ovary as is the case for 'idiopathic' PCO, or from outside the ovary, in other situations.

Follicular Arrest

The second abnormality of folliculogenesis in PCOS is the defective selection of a dominant follicle. The inhibition of the progression to the dominant follicle leads to stagnation and to the accumulation of selectable follicles, giving them their characteristic appearance of multifollicular ovaries on ultrasound. This phenomenon called 'follicular arrest' probably results from the lack of action of FSH on the excessive follicular cohort.

Is There Insufficient Secretion of FSH in PCOS?

It is a common belief that patients with PCOS have immunoreactive FSH levels at the same range as normal women in early follicular phase [16]. However, if one looks closely at all the published series, they are often slightly decreased below the 'threshold' level required during the early follicular phase to stimulate normal follicle maturation [17]. The mechanisms for this decrease are not fully elucidated. Although slightly increased E_2 levels have been reported in women with anovulatory PCOS [17], there is little evidence that they induce an excessive negative feedback. Likewise, serum inhibin B levels are not openly exaggerated in PCOS, and there is no negative correlation between serum FSH and inhibin B levels [7]. Clearly, there is still room for future investigations on that important issue.

Is There a Local Inhibition of FSH Action in PCO?

The assumption of local excess of inhibitor(s) of FSH action is based on various experimental and clinical arguments. In vitro, the GC from antral follicles of PCO produce normal and sometimes very increased amounts of estradiol in response to FSH [18], which clearly indicates that the abnormal function in vivo is not due to a lack of intrinsic action of FSH, but rather to the in vivo environment of GC which exerts an inhibitory effect. These in vitro data have been reinforced in vivo by exposure to gradually increasing doses of recombinant FSH, indicating that patients with PCOS have a response threshold in terms of production of E_2 higher than normal women [19].

So far, this partial resistance to FSH has not received a definitive explanation [17]. According to our ultrasound data, indicating a negative correlation between small (2–5 mm) and larger (6–9 mm) antral follicles [20], it is tempting to suggest a self-inhibitory effect of the cohort itself [12]. This effect would work via the secretion of factors acting locally such as anti-müllerian hormone (AMH). AMH is a member of the superfamily of TGF-β, to which belong many other proteins having a role in reproductive function. In females, AMH is detectable in GC at the end of fetal life (36 weeks) and until menopause. Its expression starts after the primary follicle differentiation, and its production varies depending on the follicular development: it is at the highest in preantral and small antral follicles and then declines in the dominant follicle [21]. Serum AMH level is strongly correlated with the number of small antral follicles; therefore, it is increased in PCOS. This is particularly useful for the diagnosis of PCO since the serum AMH assay presents itself as a very good surrogate to follicle count [22, 23]. Moreover, the increase in serum AMH in PCOS would also be due to increased production per follicle. Indeed, a four times higher production of AMH has been observed in the culture media of GC from anovulatory women with PCOS compared with normal ovulating women [24]. Similarly, the concentration of AMH in follicular fluid was significantly higher in cultured small follicles derived from PCOS compared with normal ovaries. We also showed a two times higher expression of AMH in follicles from patients with PCOS by RT-PCR [reviewed in 24].

Is the Excess of AMH a Good Candidate for Explaining Anovulation?

Physiologically, within the cohort of antral follicles, AMH is at its highest production level, and it is highly suspected to repress the FSH-dependent aromatase activity [24]. The lack of this activity has been considered for a long time as a hallmark of the 'follicular arrest' of PCOS, witnessing the lack of FSH effect [25]. In vitro studies of cultured GC from antral follicles have indicated a much higher production of AMH when they originate from anovulatory patients in comparison to normal women or ovulatory women with PCOS [24]. Therefore, in anovulatory patients, serum FSH, although at low to normal plasma concentrations, would not be able to induce a decrease in AMH sufficient to allow the expression of aromatase. In agreement, AMH plasma level is closely related to the degree of menstrual disturbance [21]. Lastly, this hypothesis was strengthened by the observation of a decrease in AMH preceding the appearance of a dominant follicle during treatment with small doses of recombinant FSH in anovulatory patients with PCOS [26].

In conclusion, the pathophysiology of PCOS cannot be summarized in a few pages as it covers many areas of gynecology, endocrinology, diabetology and nutrition. The 'fundamental' anomaly is currently unknown, but does it really exist? Would not PCOS be just a banal nonspecific ovarian response to various stimuli whose common denominator is the creation of an intraovarian hyperandrogenism? In this case, the frantic search for the 'PCOS gene', which we are currently witnessing, may frustrate many a researcher...

References

1 Norman RJ, Dewailly D, Legro RS, Hickey TE: Polycystic ovary syndrome. Lancet 2007;370:685.
2 Strauss JF III, Dunaif A: Molecular mysteries of polycystic ovary syndrome. Mol Endocrinol 1999; 13:800.
3 Taylor AE, McCourt B, Martin KA, Anderson EJ, Adams JM, Schoenfeld D, Hall JE: Determinants of abnormal gonadotropin secretion in clinically defined women with polycystic ovary syndrome. J Clin Endocrinol Metab 1997;82:2248.
4 Blank SK, McCartney CR, Helm KD, Marshall JC: Neuroendocrine effects of androgens in adult polycystic ovary syndrome and female puberty. Semin Reprod Med 2007;25:352.
5 Baptiste CG, Battista MC, Trottier A, Baillargeon JP: Insulin and hyperandrogenism in women with polycystic ovary syndrome. J Steroid Biochem Mol Biol 2010;122:42.
6 Kelly CJ, Stenton SR, Lashen H: Insulin-like growth factor binding protein-1 in PCOS: a systematic review and meta-analysis. Hum Reprod Update 2011;17:4.
7 Pigny P, Cortet-Rudelli C, Decanter C, Deroubaix D, Soudan B, Duhamel A, Dewailly D: Serum levels of inhibins are differentially altered in patients with PCOS: effects of being overweight and relevance to hyperandrogenism. Fertil Steril 2000;73:972.
8 Wickenheisser JK, Nelson-DeGrave VL, McAllister JM: Human ovarian theca cells in culture. Trends Endocrinol Metab 2006;17:65.
9 Franks S, Berga SL: Does PCOS have developmental origins? Fertil Steril 2012;97:2.
10 Hughesdon PE: Morphology and morphogenesis of the Stein-Leventhal ovary and of so-called 'hyperthecosis'. Obstet Gynecol Surv 1982;37:59.
11 Webber LJ, Stubbs S, Stark J, Trew GH, Margara R, Hardy K, Franks S: Formation and early development of follicles in the polycystic ovary. Lancet 2003;362:1017.
12 Jonard S, Dewailly D: The follicular excess in polycystic ovaries, due to intra-ovarian hyperandrogenism, may be the main culprit for the follicular arrest. Hum Reprod Update 2004;10:107.

13 Vendola KA, Zhou J, Adesanya OO, Weil SJ, Bondy CA: Androgens stimulate early stages of follicular growth in the primate ovary. J Clin Invest 1998; 101:2622.
14 Xita N, Tsatsoulis A: Review: fetal programming of polycystic ovary syndrome by androgen excess: evidence from experimental, clinical, and genetic association studies. J Clin Endocrinol Metab 2006; 91:1660.
15 Jonard S, Robert Y, Cortet-Rudelli C, Pigny P, Decanter C, Dewailly D: Ultrasound examination of polycystic ovaries: is it worth counting the follicles? Hum Reprod 2003;18:598.
16 Fauser BC, Pache TD, Lamberts SW, Hop WC, de Jong F, Dahl KD: Serum bioactive and immunoreactive luteinizing hormone and follicle-stimulating hormone levels in women with cycle abnormalities, with or without polycystic ovarian disease. J Clin Endocrinol Metab 1991;73:811.
17 Franks S, Stark J, Hardy K: Follicle dynamics and anovulation in polycystic ovary syndrome. Hum Reprod Update 2008;14:367.
18 Almahbobi G, Anderiesz C, Hutchinson P, McFarlane JR, Wood C, Trounson AO: Functional integrity of granulosa cells from polycystic ovaries. Clin Endocrinol (Oxf) 1996;44:571.
19 Coffler MS, Patel K, Dahan MH, Malcom PJ, Kawashima T, Deutsch R, Chang RJ: Evidence for abnormal granulosa cell responsiveness to FSH in women with polycystic ovary syndrome. J Clin Endocrinol Metab 2003;88:1742.
20 Dewailly D, Catteau-Jonard S, Reyss AC, Maunoury-Lefebvre C, Poncelet E, Pigny P: The excess in 2–5 mm follicles seen at ovarian ultrasonography is tightly associated to the follicular arrest of the polycystic ovary syndrome. Hum Reprod 2007;22:1562.
21 Weenen C, Laven JS, Von Bergh AR, Cranfield M, Groome NP, Visser JA, Kramer P, Fauser BC, Themmen AP: Anti-Müllerian hormone expression pattern in the human ovary: potential implications for initial and cyclic follicle recruitment. Mol Hum Reprod 2004;10:77.
22 Pigny P, Jonard S, Robert Y, Dewailly D: Serum anti-Mullerian hormone as a surrogate for antral follicle count for definition of the polycystic ovary syndrome. J Clin Endocrinol Metab 2006;91:941.
23 Dewailly D, Gronier H, Poncelet E, Robin G, Leroy M, Pigny P, Duhamel A, Catteau-Jonard S: Diagnosis of polycystic ovary syndrome (PCOS): revisiting the threshold values of follicle count on ultrasound and of the serum AMH level for the definition of polycystic ovaries. Hum Reprod 2011;26:3123.
24 Pellatt L, Rice S, Mason HD: Anti-Müllerian hormone and polycystic ovary syndrome: a mountain too high? Reproduction 2010;139:825.
25 Franks S, Mason H, White D, Willis D: Etiology of anovulation in polycystic ovary syndrome. Steroids 1998;63:306.
26 Catteau-Jonard S, Pigny P, Reyss AC, Decanter C, Poncelet E, Dewailly D: Changes in serum anti-Mullerian hormone level during low-dose recombinant follicular-stimulating hormone therapy for anovulation in polycystic ovary syndrome. J Clin Endocrinol Metab 2007;92:4138.

Didier Dewailly, MD
Service de Gynécologie Endocrinienne et Médecine de la Reproduction
Hôpital Jeanne de Flandre, CHU de Lille
2, Avenue Eugène Avinée
FR–59037 Lille Cedex (France)
Tel. +33 3 20 44 63 09, E-Mail didier.dewailly@chru-lille.fr

Macut D, Pfeifer M, Yildiz BO, Diamanti-Kandarakis E (eds): Polycystic Ovary Syndrome. Novel Insights into Causes and Therapy. Front Horm Res. Basel, Karger, 2013, vol 40, pp 28–39

Genetics of Polycystic Ovary Syndrome

Thomas M. Barber[a] · Stephen Franks[b]

[a]Division of Metabolic and Vascular Health, Warwick Medical School, University of Warwick, Coventry, and [b]Institute of Reproductive and Developmental Biology, Imperial College (Hammersmith Campus), London, UK

Abstract

Polycystic ovary syndrome (PCOS) is an oligogenic condition, with a heritability of ~70%. PCOS is also associated with obesity, which itself is heavily influenced by genetic variants. PCOS is inherently difficult to study genetically, and most of the current literature (>70 studies based on the candidate gene approach) is inconclusive, with many studies being underpowered resulting in inconsistencies, controversies and lack of clear consensus. A further problem is that the candidate gene approach relies upon some prior understanding of pathogenesis to determine the candidacy of the gene chosen (with >20,000 genes to choose from within the human genome). PCOS has a complex and incompletely understood pathogenesis, thereby limiting the candidate gene approach for this condition. Thankfully, this limitation is overcome through use of the genome-wide association study (GWAS), the first of which in PCOS has already been published. The GWAS does not rely upon any a priori understanding of pathogenesis, and as such holds the potential to reveal hitherto unexpected or even unknown pathogenic pathways that may be implicated in the development of PCOS. Data from future GWAS in PCOS should transform our understanding of PCOS pathogenesis, and also provide a basis on which to develop future novel therapeutic strategies.

Polycystic ovary syndrome (PCOS) is a genetic (likely oligogenic) condition [1], with a heritability of approximately 70% as evidenced by data derived from twin and family-based association studies, including those from a large Dutch twin-family study on >1,300 monozygotic twins and >1,800 dizygotic twins/singleton sisters of twins [2]. The pathogenesis of PCOS is influenced by an underlying genetic predisposition in addition to the effects of obesity in many women. Furthermore, obesity often unmasks PCOS-related features [3]. Environmental (particularly dietary) factors also influence the pathogenesis of PCOS through effects on body fat mass, although obesity is itself a highly heritable condition [4], raising the possibility of overlap between gene variants implicated in the susceptibility to development of PCOS and obesity per se.

Limitations Associated with Genetics Studies in PCOS

Difficulty with Retrospective Diagnosis

It is difficult to formulate an accurate retrospective diagnosis of PCOS in post-menopausal women. Ovarian morphology is an unreliable indicator of this condition after menopause, memory for menstrual pattern can be unreliable and biochemical features are variable. Unfortunately, there is no 'smoking gun' that reliably indicates a history of PCOS in post-menopausal women. In the context of a genetics study on PCOS, the assignment of affected/unaffected status to those subjects who are post-menopausal women can therefore be difficult, and this may introduce inaccuracies.

Heterogeneity

The heterogeneity of PCOS applies to many facets of the condition including menstrual cyclity, ovarian morphology, hyperandrogenic features, fertility and both endocrine and metabolic indices [1]. This heterogeneity is reflected through the use of the Rotterdam diagnostic criteria [5] in which the 'two out of three' rule that applies has led to the generation of four distinct phenotypic subgroups, with significant heterogeneity between them. We have demonstrated this in a large UK cohort, with metabolic dysfunction shown to be largely confined to those women with both hyperandrogenic features and oligo-amenorrhoea [6]. It is possible that certain gene variants implicated in susceptibility to development of PCOS associate with a particular phenotypic subgroup of the condition. Consequently, this may affect the power of a study to detect such a gene variant if an 'all-inclusive' approach is adopted for the recruitment of women with PCOS. It is important to be cognisant of the potential limitations associated with comparing genetic data between studies that used different diagnostic criteria for recruitment.

Incompletely Understood Aetiology

Any candidate gene study should be informed by some prior understanding of the aetiology of the condition being studied. The complexity and incomplete understanding of the pathogenesis of PCOS therefore presents a problem for the candidate gene study approach, which is likely to miss some important gene variants for susceptibility to development of PCOS through lack of a complete knowledge and understanding of pathogenesis. In contrast, the genome-wide association study (GWAS) approach overcomes this problem, and can reveal unexpected data that lead to novel insights into pathogenesis, the identification of *FTO* variants in a type 2 diabetes mellitus (T2D) GWAS being one such example [7].

Table 1. The limitations inherent to genetics studies in PCOS

Limitation	Problem
Difficulty with retrospective diagnosis	Inaccurate assignment of PCOS case status in post-menopausal women
Heterogeneity	Differences in diagnostic criteria between studies, and some gene effects may be restricted to certain phenotypic sub-groups
Incompletely understood aetiology	Candidate gene studies require a priori understanding of aetiology to instruct gene candidacy
Mode of inheritance and gene effect size	Relatively small gene effect sizes require larger numbers of subjects for a study to be adequately powered
Associated sub-fertility	Reduced number of offspring thereby limiting trans-generational genetics studies

Mode of Inheritance and Gene Effect Size

The effect size of the individual gene variants implicated in susceptibility to development of PCOS is likely to be small [1], requiring the inclusion of relatively large cohorts for detection. Unfortunately, much of the literature on the genetics of PCOS is littered with reports from underpowered studies, some of which claim association of a variant with PCOS only to be superseded with larger studies refuting such a claim [1]. This has confused the field somewhat and hindered progress. Future reporting of genetics studies in PCOS should be restricted to those that are adequately powered to detect the variant in question and, ideally, whose findings have been replicated in an independent cohort.

Associated Sub-Fertility

PCOS is associated with sub-fertility [8] and possibly also increased miscarriage rates [9]. These factors are likely to adversely affect trans-generational genetics studies in PCOS.

The limitations associated with genetics studies in PCOS are summarised in table 1.

Candidate Gene Studies in PCOS

Most of the reported genetics studies on PCOS in the literature have utilised a candidate gene population-based approach. The candidate gene approach has been employed to examine association of variants in >70 genes with susceptibility to development of PCOS [10]. As outlined, however, the biological significance of data from these studies is informed by the candidacy of the gene in question. With >20,000 genes in the human genome, there are plenty of genes to choose from, and it is likely that gene candidacy for PCOS will broaden as our understanding of its pathogenesis improves. In this section, we review the main candidate gene studies reported in the literature to date. To improve clarity, we have divided the section into sub-sections relating to the main components of PCOS pathogenesis.

Obesity and Insulin Resistance

Aetiology

There is a close association between obesity and PCOS, 38–88% of women with PCOS being either overweight or obese [3]. Although not a universal feature of PCOS, the development of obesity exposes or worsens the clinical, endocrine and metabolic disturbances in those women who are genetically predisposed. The heritability of obesity [4] and the overlap of obesity and PCOS, support the candidacy of gene variants that influence fat mass such as *FTO* [7] for a possible role in the susceptibility to the development of PCOS. It is likely that insulin resistance and the pleiotropic effects of hyperinsulinaemia on peripheral tissues play key roles in mediating the link between obesity and PCOS [1]. Examples include insulin acting as a co-gonadotropin on ovarian and adrenal steroidogenesis and inhibiting ovarian follicle maturation [11].

Candidate Gene Studies

In a large UK cohort (463 PCOS cases vs. >1,300 female population controls), our group published the first evidence to support genetically the established epidemiological link between obesity and PCOS. We genotyped a variant within the *FTO* gene (rs9939609) and demonstrated a significant association with PCOS status (OR 1.30 per minor allele copy) [12]. This study also provided the first evidence to support an association of a genome sequence variant with susceptibility to development of PCOS [12]. Although the effects of *FTO* variants on PCOS susceptibility are likely to be mediated via fat mass, other mechanisms cannot be excluded [12]. In a smaller study on 207 women with PCOS from a central European population, Attaoua et al. [13] demonstrated an increased prevalence of the homozygous CC genotype within *FTO* rs1421085 amongst the sub-group of women with PCOS who were also obese or who had metabolic syndrome compared with the sub-group of lean women with PCOS. In a further more recent study, it was demonstrated by Ewens et al. [14] that gene variants associated with obesity (including those in *FTO* and the Melanocortin Receptor 4 gene – *MC4R*) also contribute to an elevated BMI in PCOS, although did not appear to play an important role in the development of PCOS per se. Given the link between obesity and PCOS, it is important that other gene variants that influence fat mass are used as candidates for susceptibility to development of PCOS in future studies.

Genes encoding peroxisome proliferator-activated receptors (PPARs) including PPAR-γ are known to influence insulin sensitivity [1]. San-Millan and Escobar-Morreale [15] performed a meta-analysis on 9 candidate gene studies that examined the PPAR-γ Pro 12 Ala variant in women with PCOS, and showed a significant association of this variant with a reduced likelihood of having PCOS (OR 0.77, 95% CI 0.61–0.96, $p = 0.025$) [15]. The insulin receptor itself clearly also influences insulin sensitivity. In a study on 180 Indian women with PCOS, variants within the insulin receptor gene (*INSR*, exon 17) were shown to be associated with PCOS in the *lean* cases [16]. Another less well-known mechanism that influences insulin sensitivity includes the vitamin D pathway, with low levels of serum 25-hydroxy vitamin D having been shown to associate with obesity and insulin resistance in a cohort of 120 women with PCOS [17]. It has been demonstrated in an Iranian study on 162 women with PCOS and 162 control women that the vitamin D receptor (*VDR*) gene Apa1 polymorphism associates significantly with PCOS [18]. Given the importance of insulin resistance in the pathogenesis of PCOS, it is important to promote the candidacy of gene variants implicated in the insulin sensitivity pathway for future studies on PCOS genetics, although the studies on *INSR* and *VDR* are small, underpowered and therefore inconclusive.

β-Cell Dysfunction

Aetiology

There is substantial overlap between T2D and PCOS [3] with the risk of developing T2D being ten times that amongst women with PCOS compared with age- and BMI-matched control women [19]. This provides the rationale for choosing T2D susceptibility variants as candidates for genetic studies in PCOS. Genes known to be implicated in susceptibility for development of T2D include *TCF7L2* (encoding transcription factor 7-like 2, with a per-allele odds ratio, OR, of ~1.35) and *KCNJ11* (encoding Kir6.2 that forms the inwardly rectifying potassium channel within the β-cell membrane) [1]. The effect of common variants in *TCF7L2* and *KCNJ11* on T2D susceptibility is most likely mediated via impairment of insulin secretion from the β-cell, a well-established pathogenic pathway in T2D [20].

There is controversy in the literature regarding the role of β-cell dysfunction in the pathogenesis of PCOS [3]. It is possible to hypothesise that either reduced β-cell function (resulting in impaired glucose tolerance or hyperglycaemia) or enhanced β-cell function (resulting in hyperinsulinaemia and the resulting adverse effects on peripheral tissues outlined earlier) or even a combination may play roles in the pathogenesis of PCOS. However, regardless of whether β-cell dysfunction is implicated in the development of PCOS or the possible mechanisms involved, this does not diminish the candidacy of T2D variants as possible susceptibility variants for PCOS given the epidemiological overlap between T2D and PCOS.

Candidate Gene Studies

Our own group published data on the rs7903146 and rs12255372 variants within *TCF7L2* in a large UK cohort of women with PCOS (n = 369) versus 2,574 UK population controls, and showed no association of either variant with susceptibility to the development of PCOS or with androgen levels [21]. In support of these data, Biyasheva et al. [22] examined 58 single nucleotide polymorphisms (SNPs) mapping to *TCF7L2* in >600 PCOS cases and >550 control women, and also showed no association with PCOS, although did show an association with PCOS for two other *TCF7L2*-related SNPs mapping >100 kb centromeric to the T2D susceptibility loci. Our group also published the first candidate gene study on *KCNJ11* (E23K, a well-established T2D susceptibility variant) in PCOS. This study was based on a large UK cohort of >370 PCOS cases and >2,570 population controls, and demonstrated no association of *KCNJ11* E23K with PCOS or androgen levels.

Another gene that is relevant for insulin secretion is the insulin gene that encodes production of insulin. There is a region within the 5′ regulatory element of the insulin gene that regulates insulin gene transcription known as the variable number of tandem repeats (VNTR), which has also been shown to associate with T2D [23]. However, no evidence was shown for association of insulin gene VNTR with susceptibility to the development of PCOS in a large study involving >400 UK PCOS cases and >1,000 UK controls [23].

The data from existing candidate gene studies on T2D susceptibility variants show no convincing evidence for a genetic role of such variants in susceptibility for development of PCOS, although the existing studies are not sufficiently powered to detect subtle effects. It would appear that the genetic architecture of T2D and PCOS are qualitatively distinct, at least in terms of β-cell function. Although β-cell dysfunction plays an important role in the pathogenesis of T2D, the existing genetic evidence does not support a specific role in PCOS. In contrast, we propose that the adverse effects of insulin resistance and hyperinsulinaemia on peripheral tissues are key pathogenic factors in PCOS.

Steroid Production and Metabolism

Aetiology

Production of steroid hormones (including androgens) commences with the synthesis of cholesterol and its conversion to pregnenolone within the ovarian theca cells and adrenal cortex. This process occurs through cleavage of the P450 side chain, catalysed by the rate-limiting enzyme P450 11a1, encoded by the gene *CYP11A*. The hyperandrogenaemia of PCOS is most commonly characterised by a raised testosterone which results from enhanced ovarian biosynthesis (with variable contribution from adrenal androgens), and from peripheral conversion of the weaker androgens androstenedione (under the control of the enzyme 17β-hydroxysteroid dehydrogenase) and DHEA [3]. Peripheral conversion of testosterone into dihydrotestosterone is under the control of the enzyme, 5α-reductase, which also catabolises cortisol to affect adrenal androgen production through feedback effects [3]. In anovulatory women with PCOS, estradiol is also slightly but abnormally elevated through both enhanced ovarian granulosa cell production and peripheral aromatization of testosterone mainly within adipose tissue [3]. This is under the control of the enzyme, cytochrome P-450 aromatase, encoded by the gene *CYP19*.

Given the importance of hyperandrogenaemia to PCOS and the complexity of the steroid biosynthetic pathways, there are many potential candidate genes. Some of the main genetic studies in this field are outlined.

Candidate Gene Studies

There are some inconsistencies in the literature regarding candidate gene studies on *CYP11A* in PCOS [1]. One of the largest studies was from the UK involving >370 PCOS cases and >330 population controls and >1,500 women from the Northern Finland Birth Cohort of 1966 (NFBC1966). In this study, no association of *CYP11A* promoter allele 5 with susceptibility to development of PCOS was shown although there was an association with promoter allele 4 [24]. There is also controversy regarding a possible role for *CYP19* (encoding the aromatase enzyme) in the pathogenesis of PCOS, with one of the largest studies showing no such association [25]. Adequately powered studies are required in the future to confirm or refute possible genetic associations between *CYP11A* and *CYP19* with susceptibility to the development of PCOS. Regarding sensitivity to the steroidogenic effects of luteinizing hormone, there is some evidence that the S312N variant of the luteinizing hormone/choriogonadotropin receptor gene is implicated in susceptibility to development of PCOS in a Sardinian population [26]. This result needs to be validated in further studies.

The literature is more compelling for an important role of 5α-reductase activity in the pathogenesis of PCOS. Women with PCOS were shown convincingly to manifest increased 5α-reductase enzyme activities and adrenocortical drive compared with controls in a large UK study on 178 women with PCOS versus 100 BMI-matched controls [27]. In a study in 287 women with PCOS and 187 controls on polymorphisms within genes encoding isoforms of 5α-reductase (*SRD5A1* and *SRD5A2*), an association between haplotypes within both genes and susceptibility to development of PCOS was demonstrated [28]. Furthermore, a variant within *SRD5A2* associated with reduced activity of 5α-reductase was also associated with *protection* against the development of PCOS [28]. Again, the impact of these studies is dulled by the limitation of the relatively small cohorts studied, and further genetic studies are needed to confirm a suspected role for enhanced 5α-reductase activity in the pathogenesis of PCOS.

Androgen Receptor and X-Inactivation

Aetiology

The androgen receptor (AR), a nuclear receptor encoded by the *AR* gene located on the X-chromosome, manifests variable sensitivity to the effects of androgens and is influenced by genetic effects [1]. An important determinant of AR sensitivity is the length of a polymorphic trinucleotide (CAG) repeat sequence within exon 1 of the *AR* gene, encoding a polyglutamine tract in the N-terminal transactivation domain of the AR [1]. The length of the CAG repeat sequence within the *AR* gene influences androgenicity and therefore the development and expression of PCOS – the shorter the CAG repeat the more sensitive the AR. The pattern of X-inactivation in women also introduces the potential for epigenetic effects on *AR* gene expression and may also influence androgenicity.

Candidate Gene Studies

There are some inconsistencies in the current literature on *AR* CAG repeats in PCOS. In one of the largest studies on 330 women with PCOS and 289 controls, there was a significant 13% reduction in the odds of PCOS for each additional unit increment in the bi-allelic mean number of *AR* CAG repeats [29]. In contrast, a further study on 122 infertile women with PCOS compared with two population control groups consisting of 83 fertile women and 831 predominantly fertile Australian women demonstrated a significantly greater frequency of bi-allelic mean *AR* CAG repeat number >22 in women with PCOS compared with the two control groups [30].

A possible role for X-inactivation in PCOS development was shown in a study on 88 sisters of women with PCOS that demonstrated the same pattern of X-inactivation more frequently in sisters with the same phenotype (PCOS affected vs. unaffected status) and *AR* CAG repeat number than in sisters with different phenotypes [31]. In the study by Shah et al. [29] outlined above, it was demonstrated that amongst those women with non-random X-inactivation (>60% preferential inactivation of either allele), preferential activation of the *AR* allele with a shorter CAG repeat occurred more frequently in women with PCOS (54.3%) versus control women (46.2%; $p = 0.036$). Furthermore, in those women who had preferential activation of an *AR* allele that was shorter than the median CAG repeat length, there was a significant 2-fold increased OR of PCOS status [29].

Clearly, further large studies are required to resolve the controversy regarding the role of *AR* CAG repeat number in the pathogenesis of PCOS. The few studies on X-inactivation in PCOS do seem compelling and are consistent with what would be predicted from knowledge of CAG repeat and androgenicity. On the other hand, it is not unreasonable to conclude that variants in *AR* CAG repeats can affect expression of androgen action in women with PCOS but do not confer susceptibility to PCOS per se. It would be reassuring for the epigenetic effects of X-inactivation on the susceptibility to development of PCOS to be validated in future large studies.

Ovarian Folliculogenesis

Aetiology
One of the diagnostic criteria for PCOS is absent or irregular menses resulting from oligo-anovulation [5]. Anovulation in women with PCOS is characterised by arrested growth of antral and pre-antral follicles. Possible mechanisms include acceleration of terminal differentiation of the granulosa cells of medium-sized antral follicles (combined effects of excess of luteinizing hormone and/or insulin), or intrinsic differences in follicle development between polycystic and normal ovaries affecting both pre-antral and antral follicles [32]. Although the candidacy of genes implicated in folliculogenesis for a role in the susceptibility to development of PCOS is undoubted, the lack of candidate gene studies in this area probably reflects our incomplete understanding not only of the pathogenic pathways involved but also of the underlying physiology of ovarian follicle development.

Candidate Gene Studies
It has been demonstrated that a region of DNA on chromosome 19 (19p13.2) has a particularly strong association with susceptibility to the development of PCOS on a screen of 37 candidate genes [10, 33]. Within this region is D19S884, a dinucleotide-repeat polymorphism that maps close to *INSR* (insulin receptor gene) and intron 55 of *FBN3* (fibrillin 3 gene, the third member of the fibrillin extracellular matrix protein family) [10, 33]. Although the role of D19S884 in the development of PCOS is controversial (the finding has yet to be replicated in additional, independent, large case-control cohorts), it is possible that certain mutations in the fibrillin 3 gene (*FBN3*) may result in impaired follicle development, although this hypothesis requires genetic verification and the pathogenic mechanisms need to be explored further.

Genome-Wide Association Studies in the Context of PCOS

One problem with the candidate gene approach for studying the genetics of PCOS is that there remain many more plausible candidate loci in the human genome to choose from. This coupled with our incomplete understanding of the pathogenesis of PCOS brings credibility to the GWAS as an attractive alternative approach. A clear advantage of a GWAS is that it does not rely upon any prior understanding of candidate pathways and that the data generated may offer new insights into pathogenesis. The identification of *FTO* as a gene implicated in common obesity is a case in point [7]: no one could have predicted prior to the GWAS for T2D being performed, that a gene implicated in the fusion of toes in rodents also influences fat mass in humans. This new insight into pathogenesis would not have been possible through a candidate gene approach.

One difficulty with the GWAS approach is that due to the high number of variants being analysed, a GWAS would need to be adequately powered to detect association of certain genome sequence variants with PCOS, especially if each only has a small effect on phenotype. Typically, such studies require >2,000 PCOS probands and an equivalent number of controls in the discovery series alone, many more subjects than has previously been published on in candidate gene studies in PCOS to date. It would be difficult for a single centre to recruit this number of subjects, and for that reason GWAS are better suited to multi-centre studies that are capable of generating the numbers of subjects required to achieve a desirable level of power. Furthermore, verification of data from GWAS is required from replication cohorts. Other important factors need to be considered when executing a GWAS including the need to recruit a representative sample of population controls with adequate population stratification and avoidance of multiple ethnicities, and avoidance of over-matching of controls with cases: *FTO* would not have been identified as a gene that influences fat mass in humans in the GWAS on T2D [7] had the T2D cases and control subjects been matched for BMI: it was the difference in BMI between these two groups that revealed this important insight.

To date, there has only been one GWAS on women with PCOS reported on in the literature [34]. In this study, Chen et al. [34] demonstrated associations between PCOS and three loci: 2p16.3, 2p21 and 9q33.3. Over the next few years, there will be further GWAS reported on in PCOS. The data from these studies represent our best chance yet for identifying the gene variants implicated in susceptibility to development of PCOS that is likely to provide novel insights into the pathogenesis of this condition. Ultimately, a clear understanding of the genetics of PCOS will provide a basis on which to develop screening tools for this condition, and novel therapeutic strategies through improved understanding of pathogenesis.

Conclusions

The current literature on the genetics of PCOS is disappointing. Given that PCOS is a condition associated with obesity, it is a reasonable hypothesis that at least some of the genetic background of PCOS is related to variants that influence fat mass such as *FTO*. Evidence to support this hypothesis is outlined in this chapter, and we would expect that other fat mass-related genome sequence variants may also be demonstrated to associate with susceptibility to development of PCOS in future studies. However, it is also clear that PCOS has a complex pathogenesis and that neither are women with PCOS all obese nor do all obese women develop PCOS. Therefore, there must be other gene variants implicated that influence perhaps ovarian androgen steroidogenesis or folliculogenesis or even some hitherto unexpected or unknown process. The GWAS has the potential to shed light on novel pathogenic pathways that would otherwise have remained elusive based on conventional understanding of PCOS. The GWAS represents our best hope of identifying and understanding the genetics of PCOS, and in the process providing new insights into pathogenesis, enabling the development of new screening tests and ultimately novel therapeutic strategies. In short, the GWAS has the potential to transform our understanding and management of PCOS, and it is hugely important that future priority is given to facilitate the funding and execution of PCOS GWAS, and that the data generated are disseminated widely and form the basis for novel fields of research.

Acknowledgements

We acknowledge the many patients, relatives, nurses, and physicians who contributed to the ascertainment of the various clinical samples reported on in this chapter.

References

1 Barber TM, Franks S: Genetic basis of polycystic ovary syndrome. Exp Rev Endocrinol Metab 2010;5: 549–561.
2 Vink JM, Sadrzadeh S, Lambalk CB, Boomsma DI: Heritability of polycystic ovary syndrome in a Dutch twin-family study. J Clin Endocrinol Metab 2006;91: 2100–2104.
3 Barber TM, McCarthy MI, Wass JA, Franks S: Obesity and polycystic ovary syndrome. Clin Endocrinol (Oxf) 2006;65:137–145.
4 Lee YS: The role of genes in the current obesity epidemic. Ann Acad Med Singapore 2009;38:45–43.
5 The Rotterdam ESHRE/ASRM-sponsored PCOS consensus workshop group. Revised 2003 consensus on diagnostic criteria and long-term health risks related to polycystic ovary syndrome (PCOS). Hum Reprod 2004;19:41–47.
6 Barber TM, Wass JA, McCarthy MI, Franks S: Metabolic characteristics of women with polycystic ovaries and oligo-amenorrhoea but normal androgen levels: implications for the management of polycystic ovary syndrome. Clin Endocrinol (Oxf) 2007;66:513–517.
7 Frayling TM, Timpson NJ, Weedon MN, et al: A common variant in the FTO gene is associated with body mass index and predisposes to childhood and adult obesity. Science 2007;316:889–894.
8 Hirschberg AL: Polycystic ovary syndrome, obesity and reproductive implications. Womens Health (Lond Engl) 2009;5:529–540.
9 Koivunen R, Pouta A, Franks S, Martikainen H, Sovio U, Hartikainen AL, McCarthy MI, Ruokonen A, Bloigu A, Jarvelin MR, Morin-Papunen L: Fecundability and spontaneous abortions in women with self-reported oligo-amenorrhea and/or hirsutism: Northern Finland Birth Cohort 1966 Study. Hum Reprod 2008;23:2134–2139.
10 Urbanek M: The genetics of the polycystic ovary syndrome. Nat Clin Pract Endocrinol Metab 2007;3: 103–111.
11 Morin-Papunen LC, Vauhkonen I, Koivunen RM, Ruokonen A, Tapanainen JS: Insulin sensitivity, insulin secretion, and metabolic and hormonal parameters in healthy women and women with polycystic ovarian syndrome. Hum Reprod 2000;15: 1266–1274.
12 Barber TM, Bennett AJ, Groves CJ, et al: Association of variants in the fat mass and obesity associated (FTO) gene with polycystic ovary syndrome. Diabetologia 2008;51:1153–1158.
13 Attaoua R, Ait El Mkadem S, Radian S, Fica S, Hanzu F, Albu A, Gheorghiu M, Coculescu M, Grigorescu F: FTO gene associates to metabolic syndrome in women with polycystic ovary syndrome. Biochem Biophys Res Commun 2008;373: 230–234.
14 Ewens KG, Jones MR, Ankener W, Stewart DR, Urbanek M, Dunaif A, Legro RS, Chua A, Azziz R, Spielman RS, Goodarzi MO, Strauss JF 3rd: FTO and MC4R gene variants are associated with obesity in polycystic ovary syndrome. PLoS One 2011;6: e16390.
15 San-Millan JL, Escobar-Morreale HF: The role of genetic variation in peroxisome proliferator-activated receptors in the polycystic ovary syndrome (PCOS): an original case-control study followed by systematic review and meta-analysis of existing evidence. Clin Endocrinol (Oxf) 2010;72:383–392.
16 Mukherjee S, Shaikh N, Khavale S, Shinde G, Meherji P, Shah N, Maitra A: Genetic variation in exon 17 of INSR is associated with insulin resistance and hyperandrogenemia among lean Indian women with polycystic ovary syndrome. Eur J Endocrinol 2009;160:855–862.

17 Hahn S, Haselhorst U, Tan S, Quadbeck B, Schmidt M, Roesler S, Kimmig R, Mann K, Janssen OE: Low serum 25-hydroxyvitamin D concentrations are associated with insulin resistance and obesity in women with polycystic ovary syndrome. Exp Clin Endocrinol Diabetes 2006;114:577–583.
18 Mahmoudi T: Genetic variation in the vitamin D receptor and polycystic ovary syndrome risk. Fertil Steril 2009;92:1381–1383.
19 Legro RS, Kunselman AR, Dodson WC, Dunaif A: Prevalence and predictors of risk for type 2 diabetes mellitus and impaired glucose tolerance in polycystic ovary syndrome: a prospective, controlled study in 254 affected women. J Clin Endocrinol Metab 1999;84:165–169.
20 Rutter GA, Parton LE: The beta-cell in type 2 diabetes and in obesity. Front Horm Res 2008;36:118–134.
21 Barber TM, Bennett AJ, Groves CJ, Sovio U, Ruokonen A, Martikainen H, Pouta A, Hartikainen AL, Elliott P, Wass JA, Jarvelin MR, Zeggini E, Franks S, McCarthy MI: Disparate genetic influences on polycystic ovary syndrome (PCOS) and type 2 diabetes revealed by a lack of association between common variants within the TCF7L2 gene and PCOS. Diabetologia 2007;50:2318–2322.
22 Biyasheva A, Legro RS, Dunaif A, Urbanek M: Evidence for association between polycystic ovary syndrome (PCOS) and TCF7L2 and glucose intolerance in women with PCOS and TCF7L2. J Clin Endocrinol Metab 2009;94:2617–2625.
23 Powell BL, Haddad L, Bennett A, et al: Analysis of multiple data sets reveals no association between the insulin gene variable number tandem repeat element and polycystic ovary syndrome or related traits. J Clin Endocrinol Metab 2005;90:2988–2993.
24 Gaasenbeek M, Powell BL, Sovio U, et al: Large-scale analysis of the relationship between CYP11A promoter variation, polycystic ovarian syndrome, and serum testosterone. J Clin Endocrinol Metab 2004;89:2408–2413.
25 Gharani N, Waterworth DM, Batty S, White D, Gilling-Smith C, Conway GS, McCarthy M, Franks S, Williamson R: Association of the steroid synthesis gene CYP11a with polycystic ovary syndrome and hyperandrogenism. Hum Mol Genet 1997;6: 397–402.
26 Capalbo A, Sagnella F, Apa R, et al: The 312N variant of the luteinizing hormone/choriogonadotropin receptor gene (LHCGR) confers up to 2.7-fold increased risk of polycystic ovary syndrome in a Sardinian population. Clin Endocrinol (Oxf) 2012; 77:113–119.
27 Vassiliadi DA, Barber TM, Hughes BA, McCarthy MI, Wass JA, Franks S, Nightingale P, Tomlinson JW, Arlt W, Stewart PM: Increased 5 alpha-reductase activity and adrenocortical drive in women with polycystic ovary syndrome. J Clin Endocrinol Metab 2009;94:3558–3566.
28 Goodarzi MO, Shah NA, Antoine HJ, Pall M, Guo X, Azziz R: Variants in the 5alpha-reductase type 1 and type 2 genes are associated with polycystic ovary syndrome and the severity of hirsutism in affected women. J Clin Endocrinol Metab 2006;91: 4085–4091.
29 Shah NA, Antoine HJ, Pall M, Taylor KD, Azziz R, Goodarzi MO: Association of androgen receptor CAG repeat polymorphism and polycystic ovary syndrome. J Clin Endocrinol Metab 2008;93:1939–1945.
30 Hickey T, Chandy A, Norman RJ: The androgen receptor CAG repeat polymorphism and X-chromosome inactivation in Australian Caucasian women with infertility related to polycystic ovary syndrome. J Clin Endocrinol Metab 2002;87:161–165.
31 Hickey TE, Legro RS, Norman RJ: Epigenetic modification of the X chromosome influences susceptibility to polycystic ovary syndrome. J Clin Endocrinol Metab 2006;91:2789–2791.
32 Franks S, Stark J, Hardy K: Follicle dynamics and anovulation in polycystic ovary syndrome. Hum Reprod Update 2008;14:367–378.
33 Urbanek M, Legro RS, Driscoll DA, Azziz R, Ehrmann DA, Norman RJ, Strauss JF 3rd, Spielman RS, Dunaif A: Thirty-seven candidate genes for polycystic ovary syndrome: strongest evidence for linkage is with follistatin. Proc Natl Acad Sci USA 1999;96:8573–8578.
34 Chen ZJ, Zhao H, He L, et al: Genome-wide association study identifies susceptibility loci for polycystic ovary syndrome on chromosome 2p16.3, 2p21 and 9q33.3. Nat Genet 2011;43:55–59.

Dr. Thomas M. Barber, MA, MBBS, MRCP (UK), DPhil
Division of Metabolic and Vascular Health
Warwick Medical School, University of Warwick
Clifford Bridge Road
Coventry, CV2 2DX (UK)
E-Mail T.Barber@warwick.ac.uk

Macut D, Pfeifer M, Yildiz BO, Diamanti-Kandarakis E (eds): Polycystic Ovary Syndrome. Novel Insights into Causes and Therapy. Front Horm Res. Basel, Karger, 2013, vol 40, pp 40–50

Obesity, Adipokines and Metabolic Syndrome in Polycystic Ovary Syndrome

Enrico Carmina

Endocrine Unit, Department of Medical and Biological Sciences, University of Palermo, Palermo, Italy

Abstract

The complex mechanisms linking fat excess to metabolic syndrome are not well understood, but several experimental studies have shown that altered production of adipokines plays a main role in development and progression of this disorder. In particular, reduced secretion of adiponectin has a crucial role in inducing insulin resistance but also in determining the clustering of elevated triglycerides and small, dense LDL particles. Increased leptin secretion may be responsible for sympathetic nervous system overactivity and hypertension, while reduced omentin may have an important permissive role in the development of atherogenic processes. Finally, cytokines and other adipokines (resistin, visfatin) determine and modulate the inflammatory process that is an essential component of this condition of cardiovascular risk. Because obesity is prevalent in polycystic ovary syndrome (PCOS), it is not surprising that patients with PCOS present altered adipokine levels and increased prevalence of metabolic syndrome. However, because of the presence of other CV risk factors (androgen excess), in PCOS adipokine dysfunction is particularly severe. Understanding and treating adipokine dysfunction in young women with PCOS is an essential component of any politics of prevention of CV diseases in the general population.

Metabolic syndrome consists of the clustering in the same subject of some cardiovascular risk factors that depend on insulin resistance and abdominal obesity [1]. Because both insulin resistance and abdominal obesity are classic components of polycystic ovary syndrome (PCOS) [2], it is not surprising that, in this disorder, metabolic syndrome is much more common than in the control population [3]. In fact, also in PCOS, prevalence of metabolic syndrome is strongly correlated with the prevalence of obesity, and populations with lower bodyweight have lower prevalence of metabolic syndrome [4]. However, in women with PCOS, metabolic syndrome appears at an earlier age than in the general population, and is common also in overweight patients [1, 5]. This suggests that, in PCOS, some additional mechanisms may be important in influencing the effects of adipose tissue on the development of metabolic syndrome.

Table 1. Main adipokines and their possible role in metabolic syndrome

Adipokine	Possible physiologic role	Values in metabolic syndrome	Contribution to metabolic syndrome
Leptin	Regulation of food intake Regulation of SNS activity	Increased	Selective leptin resistance may induce overactivity of the SNS and hypertension
Adiponectin	Insulin-sensitizing hormone Protection of liver cells from negative effects of fat increase	Reduced	Low adiponectin may induce insulin resistance and altered lipid profile
Resistin	Part of the inflammatory pattern linked to adipose tissue excess	No changes	Unclear
Visfatin	Part of the inflammatory pattern linked to adipose tissue excess	Increased	Unclear
Vaspin	Regulation of food intake?	Increased	Unclear
Omentin	Protection of endothelial cells from inflammatory factors	Reduced	Low omentin levels may favor atherogenic complications of visceral fat excess
Chemerin	Regulation of adipogenesis	Increased	Unclear
RBP-4	May impair insulin sensitivity May impair liver function	Variable	Unclear
Cytokines	Part of the inflammatory pattern linked to adipose tissue excess	Increased	Atherogenic and liver complications of visceral fat excess Insulin resistance?

The complex mechanisms linking fat excess to metabolic syndrome are not well understood, but evidence is accumulating that adipokines (hormones, cytokines and other bioactive substances produced by adipose tissue) play a main role in the development of metabolic syndrome [6].

In this review, I will focus mostly on analyzing the current knowledge about adipokines and their effects on the development of metabolic syndrome in the general population. I will then discuss the special mechanisms that may be operating in women with PCOS.

Adipokines and Metabolic Syndrome in General Population

Several adipokines may be important in the development and/or progression of metabolic syndrome. In table 1, a list of main adipokines and their possible role in metabolic syndrome is given.

Leptin

Leptin is a 146-aminoacid protein which acts mostly as a signaling factor from adipose tissue to the central nervous system to serve as an indicator of energy availability [7]. Increase in fat mass leads to increased secretion of leptin and suppression of food intake. Any increase in fat mass determines an increase in serum leptin, and in general serum leptin correlates very well with total fat mass [7]. In morbid obesity, serum leptin levels are 2–4 times higher than in normal-weight subjects [7].

However, the effects of leptin on the CNS are not limited to hypothalamic regulation of appetite but involve many other cerebral areas and are essential in the regulation of energy expenditure, and glucose metabolism [7, 8]. These effects are determined by increasing sympathetic nerve activity, which in mice increases energy expenditure in interscapular brown adipose tissue.

Because the increase in serum leptin does not influence the alimentary behavior of the obese subjects, it has been suggested that, in most forms of obesity, leptin resistance develops with an unclear mechanism [7]. However, the sympathetic nervous system (SNS) is overactive in obese subjects and in metabolic syndrome [8]. Because the SNS helps regulate blood pressure, heart rate, and hepatic glucose production, selective leptin resistance may be a crucial mechanism linking increased fat mass and metabolic syndrome [8].

Adiponectin

Adiponectin, mostly the high molecular weight isoform, seems to play an important role in protecting the liver, endothelial and muscle cells from the negative effects of fat increase [9]. The activity of adiponectin is mediated by the AMP kinase system and results in enhancing cell nitric oxide (NO) production, increasing fat oxidation and inhibiting inflammatory effects.

Adiponectin is mostly produced in subcutaneous fat [10], and its values are normal or slightly low in metabolically healthy obese subjects, but are low in subjects with visceral obesity [9]. It may be one of the mechanisms that determine more severe metabolic consequences in patients with central obesity [9].

The mechanism of adiponectin decrease in subjects with visceral obesity is not clear. Some authors have suggested that the adiponectin decrease observed in obesity is the consequence of reduced insulin sensitivity and hyperinsulinemia. In fact, adiponectin circulates in inverse proportion to the degree of insulin resistance, and some data suggest that long-term changes in insulin sensitivity may downregulate adiponectin secretion. However, studies in animals have shown that adiponectin improves insulin sensitivity, and there is a growing consensus that adiponectin may be an insulin-sensitizing hormone. Instead, adiponectin decrease in visceral obesity may be the consequence of the increase in cytokines that is an important consequence of visceral obesity [11, 12].

It has been shown that patients with reduced adiponectin levels have elevated levels of small dense LDL particles [13]. Thus, the clustering of elevated triglycerides (as a result of increased large VLDL production) and small, dense LDL particles in the context of insulin resistance and obesity may be mediated by reductions of adiponectin. These data and other show that low adiponectin plays a main role in determining metabolic syndrome.

Resistin

A further adipose hormone, resistin, in animals has been linked to insulin resistance. However, human resistin is secreted by macrophages rather than adipocytes [14], and recent and growing evidence suggests that human resistin is an inflammatory biomarker that may be part of the inflammatory pattern associated with visceral obesity [14, 15].

Visfatin

This adipokine is produced by many tissues, and may have a role in promoting or maintaining systemic inflammation [15]. In fact, visfatin can induce and maintain the cellular expression of inflammatory cytokines such as TNF-α, IL-1β, and IL-6 [15].

Inside adipose tissue, visfatin is produced by differentiated adipocytes but also by the macrophages, and is part of the complex of adipose factors promoting inflammation [15]. However, the role of visfatin is probably larger, and it has been shown that visfatin may regulate β-cell function and insulin secretion.

Visfatin is increased in obesity and in metabolic syndrome, but this correlation seems to be independent of insulin resistance and mostly linked to the inflammatory pattern.

Vaspin

Vaspin is a member of the serpin (serine protease inhibitor) family that has been found increased in obesity, type 2 diabetes and metabolic syndrome [16]. However, vaspin levels increase with weight loss associated with lifestyle programs, and modifications of other adipokines (adiponectin) do not change its levels [17]. Therefore, the mean and the possible role of vaspin in obesity and metabolic syndrome are unclear.

Interestingly, it has been reported that vaspin may trigger anorectic pathways in the hypothalamus.

Omentin

Omentin is an adipokine preferentially produced by visceral adipose that circulates in two isoforms (omentin 1 and 2), with omentin-1 being the most common human circulating isoform. Omentin has an important anti-inflammatory role in the endothelium by preventing the TNF-α-induced COX-2 expression in vascular endothelial cells probably via inhibiting the JNK activation presumably through activation of AMPK/eNOS/NO pathways [18]. There is a close connection between serum omentin and adiponectin levels, and it has been suggested that regulation of omentin may be dependent on adiponectin. It is possible that omentin mediates some of the vascular effects of adiponectin.

Omentin 1 plasma levels and adipose tissue gene expression are reduced in obese and in type 2 diabetics but mostly in patients with metabolic syndrome having cardiovascular diseases [19] and in type 2 diabetes patients with carotid plaque (compared to those without carotid plaque) [20]. These data suggest an important role for omentin in determining vascular effects of metabolic syndrome.

Chemerin

Chemerin is an adipokine that regulates adipocyte development and may have some role in insulin resistance. Gene expression levels of chemerin are elevated in the adipose depots of obese compared with lean animals and markedly increase during differentiation of fibroblasts into mature adipocytes suggesting that the process of adipogenesis is in some way related to the expression or production of this adipokine.

Serum chemerin levels are elevated in patients with obesity and exhibit a positive correlation with various aspects of the metabolic syndrome [21]. It has been suggested that fasting levels of chemerin might be used as biomarker to identify insulin resistance in healthy men without typical characteristics of metabolic disorders and could be an independent predicting marker of the presence and severity of obstructive sleep apnea [22].

Retinol-Binding Protein-4

Retinol-binding protein (RBP-4) is the specific carrier protein for retinol (vitamin A) in blood and is produced by many tissues but mainly by the liver and adipose cells. It was initially hypothesized that RBP-4 may be an adipocyte signal that impairs insulin secretion. More recently, several studies have related increased production of RBP-4 to multiple risk factors for adiposity-related comorbidities. However, contrasting data exist on RBP-4 levels in obesity and metabolic syndrome, and no association with total, visceral or subcutaneous fat has been observed. In children and adolescents, serum RBP-4 correlates with liver enzymes and triglycerides and inversely with adiponectin, independent of percent body fat, suggesting a link with liver function [23].

Cytokines

Obesity, but mostly visceral obesity, is associated with chronic low-grade inflammation, and it depends in large part on increased production of different cytokines, including TNF-α, interleukin-6 and MCP-1 inside the adipose tissue [24]. In addition, cytokines, but mostly TNF-α, also seem to be important in inducing insulin resistance by impairing insulin signaling both directly by activation of serine kinases and indirectly by increasing mobilization of free fatty acids (FFA). Increased cytokine production seems to have an important role in downregulating adiponectin production in obese subjects.

Inside the adipose tissue, the cytokines are mostly produced by activated macrophages [25]. It has been suggested that the main stimulus for macrophage colonization of fat is the increased adipose cell death rate that is the consequence of adipocyte hypertrophy [25].

Adipokines and Metabolic Syndrome in General Population: Trying to Get a Full View

Mechanisms determining development and progression of metabolic syndrome are still incompletely understood. However, it is clear that in the general population the excess of adipose tissue and in particular of visceral fat is the main determinant of this risk condition. In fact, in obese subjects, insulin resistance, while essential for determining the appearance of most elements of metabolic syndrome, is only the consequence of visceral fat excess.

Most authors believe that in obese subjects insulin resistance is determined by liver accumulation of FFA released by visceral fat. However, recent evidence suggests that as adipose tissue mass expands, FFA release is downregulated, not increased [26]. The changes in adipose tissue lipolysis observed in obese subjects may simply reflect an adaptation to consistently high ambient insulin concentrations. Other mechanisms, and in particular dysfunctional regulation of adipokines, are probably more important to explain insulin resistance in the obese state.

In this respect, the reduction of adiponectin levels seems to play the main role. Because adiponectin is mainly produced in the subcutaneous fat, it has been hypothesized that increased production of cytokines inside the visceral fat is the mechanism that inhibits subcutaneous production of adiponectin. The process may be initiated by increased death of adipose cells consequent to excessive enlargement of adipose cells. It is followed by colonization and activation of macrophages and by increased

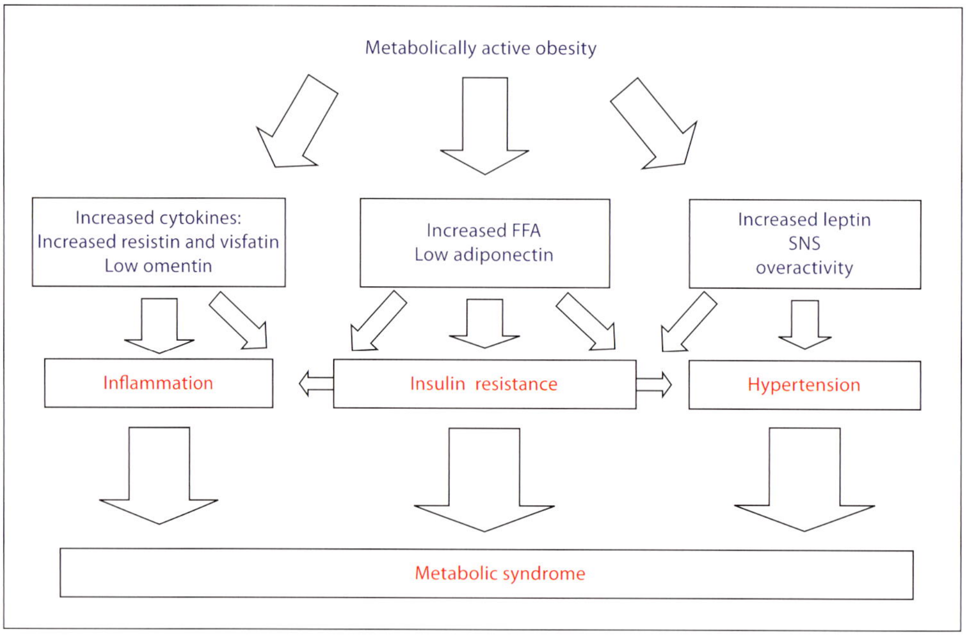

Fig. 1. Effect of adipose products on development and characteristics of metabolic syndrome.

production of several inflammatory factors, mainly cytokines but also some adipokines (resistin, visfatin).

According to some authors, impaired new adipogenesis inside visceral fat plays a pivotal role in this process. In fact, in response to the need of new adipose storage, stromal cells from the subcutaneous adipose tissue regions may proliferate and differentiate in mature adipocytes, while this process is less efficient in visceral fat depots. It probably determines differences in adipocyte size between different fat depots and increases cell death rate in visceral fat.

Several other adipokines probably participate in the development and the evolution of the metabolic syndrome. In fact, increased leptin has an important role in SNS overactivity and hypertension, while reduced omentin may have an important permissive role in the development of atherogenic process inside the cardiovascular system.

A hypothetic schematic view of the effects of adipocyte dysfunction in visceral obesity is shown in figures 1 and 2.

Adipokine Production in PCOS

Many studies have shown that adipokine secretion is altered in PCOS. However, because obesity is prevalent in this disorder, this is not surprising. As a group, patients with PCOS present higher leptin, cytokines and other inflammatory cytokines

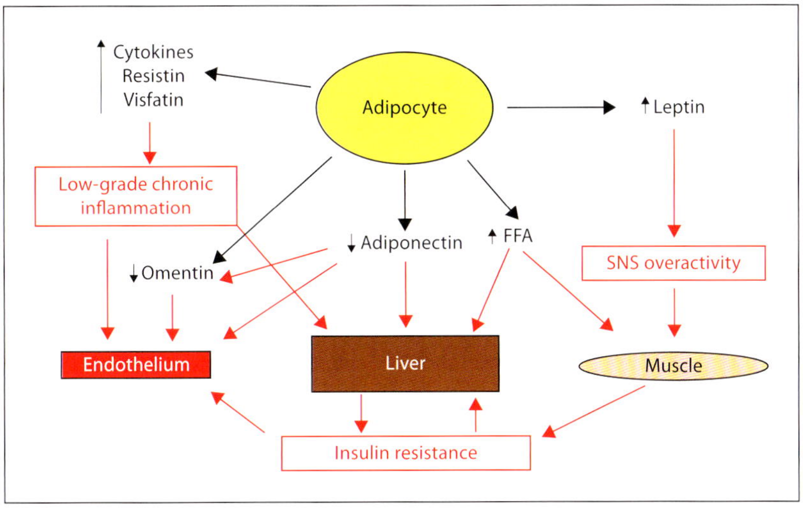

Fig. 2. Adipocyte function in metabolically active obesity.

(visfatin, vaspin, chemerin) and lower adiponectin and omentin circulating levels than the young female population.

However, when PCOS women are compared with controls matched for body-weight, some of these differences disappear, suggesting that some changes are exclusively linked to excessive adipose tissue. Many other differences remain, indicating that in PCOS adipocyte dysfunction is not only determined by the simple fat excess.

Although some discrepancy between the studies exists, probably depending on the heterogeneity of the syndrome and on differences in prevalence of obesity and fat distribution in different ethnic population, most studies have shown that, compared to weight-matched controls, women with PCOS present [26–32] (1) reduced secretion of adiponectin and omentin, (2) increased secretion of cytokines (mainly TNF-α and IL-18), visfatin, vaspin and chemerin, (3) normal secretion of leptin and resistin, (4) variable values (increased, normal, low) of RBP-4.

These findings are in large part explained by the increased prevalence of visceral (abdominal) fat in PCOS. In fact, women with PCOS present increased quantity of visceral fat not only in obese but also in overweight and in many (30–50%) normal-weight patients. Because most premenopausal obese women present increased visceral fat [2], it is not surprising that the difference in some adipocyte products is more evident in normal-weight or overweight PCOS women (compared to weight matched controls) than in obese PCOS women (compared to obese controls).

It has been shown that the same mechanisms that, in the general population, affect adipokine production are also present in women with PCOS. In fact, it has been demonstrated that also in PCOS adiponectin production in subcutaneous fat is reduced by increased secretion of cytokines by macrophages colonizing the adipose tissue.

Androgens and Adipokine Production in PCOS

Several data suggest that the adipocyte dysfunction in PCOS is not exclusively determined by increase in visceral fat. In particular, some studies have shown that the increased androgen levels that are characteristic of the syndrome may affect adipokine production and, in this way, increase prevalence and cardiovascular effects of metabolic syndrome.

The evidence that androgens influence adiponectin and adipose inflammatory factor production may be summarized as follows [33, 34]:

- While most studies evaluating total circulating adiponectin did not show any correlation between its levels and circulating androgens, it has been shown that androgen administration specifically reduces adipocyte production of HW-adiponectin, and in PCOS, HW adiponectin is negatively correlated with free testosterone levels.
- Androgens are positively correlated with TNF-α and interleukin-18 circulating levels, and androgen administration activates macrophage production of cytokines. The relationships between androgens and inflammation are complex and may be partially independent of the effects of androgens on adipose tissue. However, these data suggest that, in PCOS, increased fat production of cytokines and inflammatory adipokines is the consequence of a double mechanism involving not only increased visceral fat but also androgen activation of intra-adipose macrophages.
- While few data and some discrepancy in the results exist, it has been reported that in PCOS increased androgens are correlated with omentin reduction with a linear decrease in omentin for any quartile of free testosterone levels.

Conclusions

In PCOS, an adipocyte dysfunction exists and has a main role in determining insulin resistance and prevalence and morbidity of metabolic syndrome. This adipocyte dysfunction is the consequence of increased visceral fat in obese and non-obese subjects but also of the androgen excess that is characteristic of the disorder.

A better knowledge of the mechanisms of adipocyte dysfunction may improve our ability to treat PCOS women reducing their risk of future adverse cardiovascular events.

References

1 Carmina E: Metabolic syndrome in polycystic ovary syndrome. Min Ginecol 2006;58:109–114.
2 Carmina E, Bucchieri S, Esposito A, Del Puente A, Mansueto P, Di Fede G, Rini GB: Abdominal fat quantity and distribution in women with polycystic ovary syndrome and extent of its relation to insulin resistance. J Clin Endocrinol Metab 2007;92:2500–2505.
3 Apridonidze T, Essah PA, Iuorno MJ, Nestler JE: Prevalence and characteristics of the metabolic syndrome in women with polycystic ovary syndrome. J Clin Endocrinol Metab 2005;90:1929–1935.
4 Carmina E, Napoli N, Longo RA, Rini GB, Lobo RA: Metabolic syndrome in polycystic ovary syndrome (PCOS): lower prevalence in southern Italy than in the USA and the influence of criteria for the diagnosis of PCOS. Eur J Endocrinol 2006;154:141–145.
5 Rizzo M, Longo RA, Guastella E, Rini GB, Carmina E: Assessing cardiovascular risk in Mediterranean women with polycystic ovary syndrome. J Endocrinol Invest 2011;34:422–426.
6 Halberg N, Wernstedt-Asterholm I, Scherer PE: The adipocyte as an endocrine cell. Endocrinol Metab Clin North Am 2008;37:753–768.
7 Gautron L, Elmquist JK: Sixteen years and counting: an update on leptin in energy balance. J Clin Invest 2011;121:2087–2093.
8 Enriori PJ, Sinnayah P, Simonds SE, Garcia Rudaz C, Cowley MA: Leptin action in the dorsomedial hypothalamus increases sympathetic tone to brown adipose tissue in spite of systemic leptin resistance. J Neurosci 2011;31:12189–12197.
9 Guerre-Millo M: Adiponectin: an update. Diabetes Metab 2008;34:12–18.
10 Carmina E, Chu MC, Moran C, Tortoriello D, Vardhana P, Tena G, Preciado R, Lobo R: Subcutaneous and omental fat expression of adiponectin and leptin in women with polycystic ovary syndrome. Fertil Steril 2008;89:642–648.
11 Matsuzawa Y: Adiponectin: a key player in obesity related disorders. Curr Pharm Des 2010;16:1896–1901.
12 Cook JR, Semple RK: Hypoadiponectinemia – cause or consequence of human 'insulin resistance'? J Clin Endocrinol Metab 2010;95:1544–1554.
13 Weiss R, Otvos JD, Flyvbjerg A, Miserez AR, Frystyk J, Sinnreich R, Kark JD: Adiponectin and lipoprotein particle size. Diabetes Care 2009;32:1317–1319.
14 Schwartz DR, Lazar MA: Human resistin: found in translation from mouse to man. Trends Endocrinol Metab 2011;22:259–265.
15 Curat CA, Wegner V, Sengenes C, Miranville A, Tonus C, Busse R, Bouloumie A: Macrophages in human visceral adipose tissue: increased accumulation in obesity and a source of resistin and visfatin. Diabetologia 2006;49:744–747.
16 Choi SH, Kwak SH, Lee Y, Moon MK, Lim S, Park YJ, Jang HC, Kim MS: Plasma vaspin concentrations are elevated in metabolic syndrome in men and are correlated with coronary atherosclerosis in women. Clin Endocrinol (Oxf) 2011;75:628–635.
17 Kim SM, Cho GJ, Yannakoulia M, Hwang TG, Kim IH, Park EK, Mantzoros CS: Lifestyle modification increases circulating adiponectin concentrations but does not change vaspin concentrations. Metabolism 2011;60:1294–1299.
18 Yamawaki H, Kuramoto J, Kameshima S, Usui T, Okada M, Hara Y: Omentin, a novel adipocytokine inhibits TNF-induced vascular inflammation in human endothelial cells. Biochem Biophys Res Commun 2011;408:339–343.
19 Shang FJ, Wang JP, Liu XT, Zheng QS, Xue YS, Wang B, Zhao LY: Serum omentin-1 levels are inversely associated with the presence and severity of coronary artery disease in patients with metabolic syndrome. Biomarkers 2011;16:657–662.
20 Yoo HJ, Hwang SY, Hong HC, Choi HY, Yang SJ, Seo JA, Kim SG, Kim NH, Choi KM, Choi DS, Baik SH: Association of circulating omentin-1 level with arterial stiffness and carotid plaque in type 2 diabetes. Cardiovasc Diabetol 2011;22:103.
21 Ernst MC, Sinal CJ: Chemerin: at the crossroads of inflammation and obesity. Trends Endocrinol Metab 2010;21:660–667.
22 Feng X, Li P, Zhou C, Jia X, Kang J: Elevated levels of serum chemerin in patients with obstructive sleep apnea syndrome. Biomarkers 2012;17:248–253.
23 Conroy R, Espinal Y, Fennoy I, Accacha S, Boucher-Berry C, Carey DE, Close S, DeSantis D, Gupta R, Hassoun AA, Iazzetti L, Jacques FJ, Jean AM, Michel L, Pavlovich K, Rapaports R, Rosenfeld W, Shamoon E, Shelov S, Speiser PW, Ten S, Rosenbaum M: Retinol binding protein 4 is associated with adiposity-related co-morbidity risk factors in children. J Pediatr Endocrinol Metab 2011;24:913–919.
24 Lumeng CN, Saltiel AR: Inflammatory links between obesity and metabolic disease. J Clin Invest 2011;121:2111–2117.
25 Samaan MC: The macrophage at the intersection of immunity and metabolism in obesity. Diabetol Metab Syndr 2011;3:29.

26 Carmina E, Orio F, Palomba S, Cascella T, Longo RA, Colao AM, Lombardi G, Lobo RA: Evidence for altered adipocyte function in polycystic ovary syndrome. Eur J Endocrinol 2005;152:389–394.
27 Sathyapalan T, Atkin SL: Mediators of inflammation in polycystic ovary syndrome in relation to adiposity. Mediators Inflamm 2010;2010:758656.
28 Carmina E, Bucchieri S, Mansueto P, Rini G, Ferin M, Lobo RA: Circulating levels of adipose products and differences in fat distribution in the ovulatory and anovulatory phenotypes of polycystic ovary syndrome. Fertil Steril 2009;91:1332–1335.
29 Tan BK, Adya R, Farhatullah S, Lewandowski KC, O'Hare P, Lehnert H, Randeva HS: Omentin-1, a novel adipokine, is decreased in overweight insulin-resistant women with polycystic ovary syndrome: ex vivo and in vivo regulation of omentin-1 by insulin and glucose. Diabetes 2008;57:801–808.
30 Tan BK, Chen J, Digby JE, Keay SD, Kennedy CR, Randeva HS: Increased visfatin messenger ribonucleic acid and protein levels in adipose tissue and adipocytes in women with polycystic ovary syndrome: parallel increase in plasma visfatin. J Clin Endocrinol Metab 2006;91:5022–5028.
31 Tan BK, Heutling D, Chen J, Farhatullah S, Adya R, Keay SD, Kennedy CR, Lehnert H, Randeva HS: Metformin decreases the adipokine vaspin in overweight women with polycystic ovary syndrome concomitant with improvement in insulin sensitivity and a decrease in insulin resistance. Diabetes 2008;57:1501–1507.
32 Tan BK, Chen J, Farhatullah S, Adya R, Kaur J, Heutling D, Lewandowski KC, O'Hare JP, Lehnert H, Randeva HS: Insulin and metformin regulate circulating and adipose tissue chemerin. Diabetes 2009;58:1971–1977.
33 Xu A, Chan KW, Hoo RL, Wang Y, Tan KC, Zhang J, Chen B, Lam MC, Tse C, Cooper GJ, Lam KS: Testosterone selectively reduces the high molecular weight form of adiponectin by inhibiting its secretion from adipocytes. J Biol Chem 2005;280:18073–18080.
34 González F: Inflammation in polycystic ovary syndrome: underpinning of insulin resistance and ovarian dysfunction. Steroids 2012;77:300–305.

Enrico Carmina, MD
Endocrine Unit, Department of Medical and Biological Sciences, University of Palermo
Via delle Croci 47
IT–90139 Palermo (Italy)
Tel. +39 091 332377, E-Mail enrico.carmina@ae-society.org

Macut D, Pfeifer M, Yildiz BO, Diamanti-Kandarakis E (eds): Polycystic Ovary Syndrome. Novel Insights into Causes and Therapy. Front Horm Res. Basel, Karger, 2013, vol 40, pp 51–63

Dyslipidemia and Oxidative Stress in PCOS

Djuro Macut[a] · Jelica Bjekić-Macut[b] · Ana Savić-Radojević[c]

[a]Clinic for Endocrinology, Diabetes and Metabolic Diseases, [b]CHC Bežanijska kosa, [c]Institute of Medical and Clinical Biochemistry, Faculty of Medicine, University of Belgrade, Belgrade, Serbia

Abstract

Polycystic ovary syndrome (PCOS) is a common metabolic and reproductive disorder in women. An increased cardiovascular risk has to be anticipated in PCOS as it is a metabolically unstable condition. Among cardiovascular risk factors, dyslipidemia is certainly the most persistent and highly prevalent. Predominant observation is an elevation of LDL cholesterol in all PCOS patients. Decreased concentrations of HDL cholesterol are found in obese PCOS from the third decade of life onwards while triglycerides start to rise from the second decade of life. PCOS is associated with oxidative stress, namely increased production of free radicals followed by decreased serum antioxidant levels and antioxidant enzyme activity. Broad range of endocrine and metabolic disturbances like obesity, hyperinsulinemia as well as dyslipidemia might be responsible for PCOS-associated oxidative stress. Therapeutic interventions in PCOS women based on lifestyle modification as well as use of insulin sensitizers did not show significant effect on dyslipidemia. Statins are considered to be a group of promising agents that are safe and effective in improving total cholesterol, LDL cholesterol and triglycerides, and possess antioxidant activity. Supplementation with omega-3 fatty acids, α-lipoic acid and N-acetylcysteine is considered to have an anti-inflammatory and antioxidant effect and to improve dyslipidemia and insulin sensitivity in PCOS women.

Polycystic ovary syndrome (PCOS) is considered to be the most common endocrine disorder among women of reproductive age and a cause of chronic anovulation. Central features of the metabolic disturbance are peripheral insulin resistance and hyperinsulinemia, and together with centripetal fat distribution, constitute a cluster of risk factors for development of cardiovascular disease that has been a major concern for the long-term management of women with PCOS. Disturbances in lipid and lipoprotein metabolism are fairly common in women with PCOS [1]. However, interpreting the relevance of these abnormalities in terms of cardiovascular risk is complicated by inconsistencies among studies on the assessment of dyslipidemia, and by unknown mechanism how the combined risk factors translate into a real risk of developing cardiovascular disease.

Oxidative stress was recognized as one of the predisposing factors for the development of cardiovascular disease. It could be a missing link for the unfavorable metabolic conditions such as obesity and diabetes to accumulate dysfunctional proteins, lipid peroxidation products and damaged nuclear or mitochondrial DNA. PCOS is associated with oxidative stress and increased production of free radicals followed by decreased serum total antioxidant levels [2]. It is supposed that a broad range of endocrine and metabolic disturbances like obesity, hyperinsulinemia as well as dyslipidemia might be responsible for PCOS-associated oxidative stress.

Lipid Changes in Women with PCOS

Prevalence of Dyslipidemia in PCOS

Dyslipidemia is the most common metabolic abnormality in PCOS, although the type and extent of the derangement has been variable. According to the National Cholesterol Education Program guidelines, about 70% of PCOS women have borderline or high lipid levels [1].

Ethnicity could represent an important determinant of the metabolic derangements in population. A recent Danish study on a significant number of women with PCOS showed differences for the median values of total cholesterol, LDL cholesterol and triglycerides, although obtained lipid values were within the range of normality [3].

Family history of dyslipidemia is often present in PCOS subjects. The relative risk for developing dyslipidemia is estimated to be 1.8 in PCOS family members [4]. Elevated triglycerides are present in pubertal period in daughters of PCOS women, even before the onset of hyperandrogenism. In PCOS women that have a positive family history on the PCOS-related clinical abnormality, higher values of total cholesterol, LDL cholesterol, Apo B and triglycerides were found [5].

Pathophysiology of Dyslipidemia in PCOS

Influence of Aging and Body Composition

Lipid abnormalities were found in women with PCOS from their fourth decade of life [6]. This gave us the clue towards the existence of an increased cardiovascular risk over a lifetime in these women. A flat slope of increasing total cholesterol and LDL cholesterol with age in PCOS women was observed in comparison with controls who showed a slow increase with age. Even younger obese subjects with PCOS showed aggravation in assessed cardiovascular risk factors with transition from the second to the third decade of life, giving the youngest PCOS population a potential to develop cardiovascular disease later in life [7].

Obesity affects over 50% of women with PCOS. Both non-obese and obese PCOS phenotypes are prone to increase waist-to-hip ratio, have abdominal obesity, and are consequently more susceptible to develop dyslipidemia [1]. Protein kinase A-hormone-sensitive lipase complex activity was shown to be markedly increased in visceral fat cells isolated from young women with PCOS. This was caused by changes at the post-adrenoreceptor level without alterations in the antilipolytic properties of visceral fat cells [4]. Therefore, controlling for the confounder of obesity has become the standard for analysis of lipids in PCOS women.

Influence of Hyperandrogenemia

The relation of hyperandrogenism and lipid metabolism is still not fully understood. It was shown that prolonged testosterone stimulation induces insulin resistance mediated by androgen receptor that is independent of phosphatidylinositol 3-kinase activation in adipose tissue. Testosterone acts mainly through upregulation of two genes involved in the catabolism of HDL, scavenger receptor B1 and hepatic lipase (HL). However, correlation between testosterone levels and HL activity was not confirmed in women with PCOS [8]. Androgens decrease catabolic removal of LDL by attenuating estrogen receptor-mediated induction of LDL receptor activity. Androgens as other sex steroids regulate lipoprotein lipase (LPL) activity in humans. In obese women postprandial LPL activity correlates positively with plasma-free testosterone, while there is an inverse relation between testosterone and LPL activity in adipose tissue of PCOS women [4].

Influence of Insulin Resistance

PCOS women with impaired glucose tolerance or type 2 diabetes had significantly greater prevalence of lipid abnormalities in comparison to PCOS women with normal glucose tolerance (88 vs. 58%). Accordingly, of those PCOS with insulin resistance, 81% demonstrated lipid abnormalities compared with 65% of those with normal insulin sensitivity. Hepatic overproduction of apolipoprotein B-containing VLDL seems to be the crucial mechanism linking insulin resistance and hypertriglyceridemia. Low HDL levels are frequently associated with hypertriglyceridemia in insulin-resistant states. Women with PCOS have significantly lower levels of HDL cholesterol, a strong metabolic predictor of coronary heart disease [1].

Common Lipid Disturbances in PCOS

Total Cholesterol, LDL Cholesterol Subfractions and Lipoprotein(a)

The predominant observation of most studies in women with PCOS was an elevation of LDL cholesterol in both lean and obese patients. However, a simple quantitative measurement of LDL concentration may be misleading since LDL does not exist as homogenous particles. LDL particles that are small and dense (LDL-III and LDL-IV) are considered to be more atherogenic than larger buoyant LDL species (LDL-I and LDL-II). Presence of small LDL particles, even with normal LDL cholesterol concentrations, is associated with a higher incidence of coronary artery disease (CAD). Milder forms of atherogenic dyslipidemia, namely lower total cholesterol, LDL cholesterol as well as lower levels of small, dense LDL particles, were found in ovulatory in comparison to anovulatory PCOS subgroups. A recent analysis of lipid particle profile in PCOS women using polyacrylamide gel tube electrophoresis revealed that HDL, LDL or triglyceride concentrations did not differ from controls. However, PCOS women had higher levels of VLDL, and were more likely to have an atherogenic LDL particle size pattern with small-dense LDL particles. It was found that the presence of PCOS per se was the most important determinant for the probability of having atherogenic LDL pattern [9]. Correlation of LDL particle size and decreased SHBG as a marker of androgen excess, could lead to the conclusion that androgen excess may have an early modifying effect on LDL size in women with PCOS [8], although decreased SHBG production is also a consequence of insulin resistance.

Metabolic transformation of LDL cholesterol by increased oxidation leads to higher atherogenic potential of modified LDL particles. It is known that patients with CAD have elevated levels of oxidized LDL (OxLDL), therefore establishing OxLDL as a potential novel marker of atherosclerosis. Recently, OxLDL was found to be elevated in both non-obese and obese phenotypes of PCOS and suggested to be a marker of an altered lipid metabolism and early atherosclerosis in those women [10].

Lipoprotein(a), Lp(a), represents a specific heterogeneous class of lipoprotein particles that is metabolically distinct from LDL, genetically determined, and remains stable during lifetime. Aside from LDL cholesterol, HDL cholesterol and triglycerides, Lp(a) without other apolipoproteins or lipid subfractions, provides a substantial prediction for coronary heart disease and stroke giving higher relative risk to the women than men. It was found that 24% of PCOS women had significantly higher Lp(a) concentrations, and suggested that measurement of Lp(a) in those women could be used for the assessment of cardiovascular risk and treatment goals [11].

Significance of HDL Cholesterol in PCOS

It was demonstrated that women with PCOS had significantly lower levels of HDL cholesterol, a particle that was thought to be the strongest metabolic predictor of coronary heart disease [6]. Although some investigators described higher HDL cholesterol levels than normal, this difference was not significant after adjusting for BMI and fasting insulin [1]. It was suggested that PCOS selectively reduced HDL. HL and phospholipid transfer protein remove lipid from HDL, and are induced by obesity and consequent insulin resistance [7]. Higher levels of HDL cholesterol were found in overweight and obese African-American women in comparison to Caucasian women with PCOS that were equal in BMI and insulin resistance. This is an apparent paradox as it is considered that African-American women overall have higher cardiovascular mortality than Caucasians. These observations raise the question about whether current HDL cholesterol cutoff points may inappropriately exclude some high-risk individuals from a diagnosis of metabolic syndrome (MetSy) even though their actual cardiovascular risk warrants it. Therefore, it was suggested that there may be racial differences in HDL cholesterol at least in PCOS women, which could affect cardiovascular risk classification [12].

Besides potential racial differences, variations in HDL cholesterol concentration have to be evaluated in relation to the age and BMI of patients, and in the light of compositional derangements of HDL in PCOS women. Decreased levels of total HDL were observed from the third, and of the HDL2 subfraction from the fourth decade of life [6]. Decrease in HDL was also confirmed after adjusting for age, BMI and waist circumference [13].

Triglycerides in Metabolic Derangements of PCOS
Elevated triglycerides represent a common and consistent lipid disturbance in women with PCOS [6, 7, 8, 13] starting to appear in the second decade of life, and have been found in both younger and older groups [6]. Furthermore, PCOS women with family history of menstrual abnormality and type 2 diabetes had higher triglyceride levels [5].

MetSy in patients with PCOS most frequently included atherogenic dyslipidemia characterized by elevated serum triglycerides, increased LDL particle number, and decreased HDL cholesterol levels. The prevalence of low HDL cholesterol was 42% and of elevated triglycerides 32% in PCOS patients having MetSy. Furthermore, when the top decile cutoff points for CAD risk factors were established, white women with PCOS were significantly more likely to have top decile triglycerides in comparison to respective controls (31 vs. 19%) [13].

Various lipid ratios can be used as useful tools for the assessment of metabolic and cardiovascular risk. Lipid accumulation product (LAP) represents a novel surrogate cardiovascular risk factor calculated from fasting triglycerides and waist circumference. LAP is a simple index for the assessment of visceral fat accumulation in adults, and a better indicator than BMI for identifying adults at cardiovascular risk. LAP is higher in PCOS women and related to insulin resistance and impaired glucose tolerance. Hence, LAP may reflect increased cardiovascular risk resulting from the central lipid accumulation that is frequently observed in PCOS [14]. Other proatherogenic lipid ratios highly predictive of cardiovascular risk like Apo B:Apo A1, total cholesterol:HDL cholesterol, LDL cholesterol:HDL cholesterol, and triglyceride:HDL cholesterol were significantly higher in PCOS [15].

It is suggested that postprandial triglyceride response has a role in the development of CAD. Postprandial lipemia may increase an uptake of triglyceride-rich remnants by endothelial cells, and thus increasing atherogenic intracellular accumulation of cholesterol esters. Even non-obese PCOS women were shown to have higher postprandial triglyceride response suggesting the existence of an intrinsic lipid abnormality in those women in the absence of obesity [8].

Oxidative Stress and PCOS

Oxidative stress has been recognized in various pathological disorders, such as obesity, diabetes, cardiovascular disease and atherogenesis. It is the pathologic condition in which the balance of oxidant generation and detoxification is tipped toward a pro-oxidant state, namely overwhelming an antioxidant defense and leading to accumulation of reactive oxygen species (ROS) [16].

The enumerated ROS can be converted to extremely aggressive substances that oxidize practically all cellular components. Polyunsaturated fatty acid constituents in lipids are highly vulnerable to oxidation, resulting in formation of different lipid radicals. This lipid peroxidation can damage membrane integrity and consequently impair cellular compartmentalization. In the proteins, different amino acid residues, but principally the sulfhydryl (–SH) groups, are the target of oxidation, causing changes in protein activity and selective degradation [17], thus damaging cellular function and, in extreme cases, destroying the cell. Although ROS and reactive nitrogen species are short-lived molecules, they are detectable through modified oxidative products such as nitrated tyrosines, protein carbonyls and oxidized thiol groups. Isoprostanes, malondialdehyde, and 4-hydroxyl-2-nonenol are remnant signs of lipid peroxidation, while 8-hydroxy-2′-deoxyguanosine is a marker of DNA oxidation.

PCOS is associated with oxidative stress in which increased production of free radicals is followed by decreased serum total antioxidant levels [2]. Furthermore, it has been shown that even lean women with PCOS exhibit increased oxidative stress [18, 19].

Potential Sources of Free Radicals in PCOS

Adipose Tissue

The increase in obesity-associated oxidative stress is probably due to the presence of excessive adipose tissue itself, because adipocytes and preadipocytes have been identified as a source of proinflammatory cytokines that are potent stimulators of the production of reactive oxygen and nitrogen species. Adipose tissue also has the secretory capacity of angiotensin II, which stimulates nicotinamide adenine dinucleotide phosphate (NADPH) oxidase activity. Thus, NADPH oxidase comprises the major route for ROS production in adipocytes [20].

Fatty Acid Oxidation

In vitro studies have shown that saturated fatty acids regulate expression of chemotactic factors in cultured adipose cells by mechanism that involves ROS generation and activation of cells responsible for innate immunity (mononuclear cells – MNCs). Metabolic burden of fat intake appears to be responsible for oxidative stress and insulin resistance, regardless of whether obesity is present. Namely, mitochondrial and peroxisomal oxidation of fatty acids in the liver, as well as, stimulation of NADPH oxidase activity in response to saturated fatty acids in muscle cells are suggested to be responsible for increased production of ROS [20].

Hyperglycemia

It is well established that hyperglycemia induces overproduction of ROS, especially superoxide and peroxynitrite radicals. Namely, hyperglycemia induces increased activities of both NADPH oxidase and inducible nitric oxide (NO) synthase, accelerating nonenzymatic formation of advanced glycation end products. However, it has also been shown that the activation of these ROS production pathways is secondary to the generation of free radicals at the level of the mitochondria during high glucose overload, which result in altered cellular redox state. Besides confirmed role in gene transcription of proinflammatory molecules, hyperglycemia-induced ROS production affects the activity of redox-sensitive signaling pathways, such as the phosphatidylinositol 3-kinase-phosphoinositide-dependent kinase-1-protein kinase B (Akt) signaling axis, which is involved in pleiotropic biological actions of insulin [21].

Enzymatic Sources of Free Radicals in PCOS

It can be assumed that the major enzymatic source of free radicals in PCOS is NADPH oxidase of MNCs, which lead to increased production of superoxide radicals in response to both hyperglycemia and increased levels of free fatty acids. Adipose tissue, especially in the abdominal region, may perpetuate the hyperglycemia-induced oxidative stress to promote altered TNFα release from MNCs in obese women with PCOS. Increased NADPH oxidase expression and subsequent ROS generation may, in turn, promote the insulin resistance observed in obese women with PCOS. Besides the MNCs expressing NADPH oxidase, different isoforms of NADPH oxidase can also be found in the endothelium, fibroblasts, vascular smooth muscle cells, and myocardial cells. These cardiovascular forms of enzyme are suggested to be major intrinsic sources of ROS both in the heart and in vascular tissues, and are strongly associated with atherosclerosis and hypertension [2].

Recently, an increased activity of another ROS-producing enzyme, xanthine oxidase that consumes molecular oxygen (O_2) and produces superoxide radical and hydrogen peroxide (H_2O_2), has been shown in PCOS women [19]. Hence, upregulated endothelial xanthine oxidase may also be an important source of free radicals in PCOS.

Nitric Oxide in PCOS

NO was extensively studied in PCOS. The most important source of the short-lived but rapidly diffusible NO is the endothelium. NO synthase uses L-arginine and NADPH to produce NO in the presence of tetrahydrobiopterin as an electron carrier. However, in the absence of either L-arginine or tetrahydrobiopterin, the enzyme generates superoxide radical and H_2O_2. Under oxidative stress conditions, the interaction of NO and ROS results in the production of peroxynitrite and other reactive NO species, all of which are oxidizing agents. Therefore, NO is considered harmful and useful at the same time. The so-called 'good NO' is a ROS scavenger, can prevent lipid peroxidation, and as mediator has several beneficial effects against oxidative injury. It is a vasorelaxing factor that restores blood flow, inhibits neutrophil and leukocyte adhesion and activation, limits the ROS production of NADPH oxidase, and inhibits platelet aggregation. NO can decrease LDL oxidation as well.

Insulin signal transduction pathway normally induces NO production in vascular endothelium, but in insulin-resistant states, such as PCOS, endothelial NO release is impaired [18]. Under oxidative stress conditions, formation of peroxynitrite radical ($ONOO^-$), as a result of reaction between superoxide and NO, is responsible for nitration of tyrosine residues in proteins. Therefore, presence of nitrotyrosine in plasma proteins is considered as indirect evidence of $ONOO^-$ production. Reaction of lipids with $ONOO^-$ leads to peroxidation (malondialdehyde and conjugated diene formation) and formation of nitrated lipid oxidation adducts. $ONOO^-$ can inhibit superoxide dismutase (SOD), glutaredoxin and other antioxidant molecules and systems leading to positive feedback cycles of intracellular oxidant generation and exacerbation of the oxidative cellular injury.

Mitochondrial Dysfunction in PCOS

Mitochondria are the site where the largest amounts of ROS are generated, causing defects in mitochondrial metabolism. Impairment of mitochondrial function in PCOS has been addressed recently. It was suggested that complex I of the electron transport chain is a target of the ROS that is generated in PCOS, causing a decrease in the mitochondrial consumption of O_2 and subsequent increase in the ROS production, TNFα levels, and the ratio of oxidized to reduced form of glutathione (GSSG:GSH) [22].

Until now, evidence on oxidative stress in PCOS has been based on increased plasma lipid (malondialdehyde, isoprostanes) and protein oxidative damage (SH groups) [2, 18, 19]. Our recent results on increased plasma nitrotyrosine levels appear to be the first evidence of nitrosative damage of plasma proteins in insulin-resistant patients with PCOS [19]. Women with PCOS exhibit increased ROS generation in response to both hyperglycemia and free fatty acids that is independent of obesity. The resultant oxidative stress induces a proinflammatory state that may contribute to the insulin resistance and hyperandrogenism in PCOS.

Endogenous Defense Mechanisms against ROS

It is questioned whether increased generation of ROS in PCOS is the primary event, and how the antioxidant enzymes are involved. Recyclable or replaceable sacrificial molecules can scavenge ROS in order to prevent the damage of vital biomolecules by buffering the oxidants. Some can even restore oxidized constituents, thus preventing or reducing oxidative cell injury. These substances are typically crucial elements of intermediary metabolism and therefore are naturally occurring molecules. Ascorbic acid, tocopherols, carotenoids, uric acid, ubiquinone, bilirubin, glutathione, metallothioneins and albumin are natural scavengers or nonenzymatic antioxidants [17].

Besides nonenzymatic antioxidant system, the major antioxidant enzymes are SOD, catalase and glutathione peroxidase (GPX). SOD and GPX act in a mutually supportive fashion to remove excess of superoxide, H_2O_2 and other lipid peroxides. SOD converts superoxide anions to H_2O_2, which is further reduced to water molecules by the activity of GPX [17].

When obesity persists for a long time, antioxidant sources can be depleted, decreasing the activity of antioxidant enzymes. Recently, it has been shown that in animal model of obesity, overexpression of GPX diminishes proinflammatory gene expression and ameliorates insulin resistance [23]. Therefore, considering the role of GPX in maintaining the bioavailability of vascular NO, the use of plasma GPX was highlighted as a potential target for intervention in insulin resistance states.

In PCOS women, serum total antioxidant status, which combines the concentrations of individual antioxidants such as vitamin C, E, β-carotene and thiol groups, is decreased [24]. Still, the data on key enzymatic components of plasma antioxidant system are limited and inconsistent, and have to be estimated in oxidative imbalance in PCOS.

From Oxidative Stress to Insulin Resistance

Insulin resistance is observed in both non-obese and obese women with PCOS. The molecular basis for insulin resistance, though not yet fully understood, may be related to a postreceptor defect involving oxidative stress-mediated serine and threonin (Ser/Thr) phosphorylation of the insulin receptor substrates 1 and 2 (IRS-1, IRS-2), which leads to an abrogation of insulin signaling. Specifically, serine-phosphorylated IRS molecules lose efficacy in binding to the insulin receptor that leads to impaired insulin action with compensatory hyperinsulinemia. Furthermore, when Ser/Thr phosphorylated, IRS molecules are more susceptible to proteasomal degradation. The alterations in IRS function and integrity result in impaired metabolic effects of insulin, particularly with respect to glucose transport with paradoxical persisting mitogenic effects of insulin. In fact, certain mitogenic pathways, including those involving the mitogen-activated protein kinase (MAPK), are activated in PCOS and may potentiate the resistance to insulin since MAPK activity leads to Ser/Thr phosphorylation of IRS-1 [25].

When glucose and free fatty acid levels increase, an oxidative stress is caused along with activation of stress-sensitive signaling pathways. In turn, activation of these pathways worsens both insulin action and secretion. Consequently, insulin-resistant patients, with and without type 2 diabetes, are at increased risk for developing the MetSy, a major cause of heart disease [25].

Consequences of Oxidative Stress in PCOS

Although PCOS was established as a condition with oxidative stress, the mechanisms by which free radicals are contributing to metabolic and endocrine disorders in this syndrome still remain elusive. Oxidative stress originating from glucose-activated MNCs, recruited into the polycystic ovary, may induce a local inflammatory response that stimulates ovarian androgen production in women with PCOS. Recent evidence suggests that both proinflammatory cytokines and oxidative stress may play a role in the dysregulation of the theca-interstitial compartment. Oxidative stress may have dual effect on theca cells. More pronounced oxidative stress as well as antioxidants (i.e. vitamin E succinate) inhibit proliferation of theca cells, while modest oxidative stress stimulates their proliferation in vitro [26]. In addition to stimulating proliferation of theca cells, moderate oxidative stress also induces testosterone and progesterone production by enhancing thecal expression of key steroidogenic enzymes, such as CYP17, CYP11A1, and 3βHSD. In contrast, in vitro studies have shown an inhibition of ovarian steroidogenic enzymes by antioxidants such as statins. Thus, the excess androgen production in PCOS is not only due to increased number of theca cells, but also to an induction of their steroidogenic capacity. Furthermore, oxidative stress impairs insulin signaling resulting in a compensatory hyperinsulinemia, which, in turn, further stimulates thecal steroidogenesis. Overall, PCOS involves oxidative stress with systemic inflammation, insulin resistance and consequent hyperinsulinemia that all promote dysregulation of the ovarian thecal compartment and dysfunction of endothelial cells, and result in hyperandrogenism, anovulation, and cardiovascular disorders [27]. Complex interrelation of oxidative stress and dyslipidemia as related to metabolic and cardiovascular consequences of PCOS is given in figure 1.

Therapeutic Modalities for Dyslipidemia and Oxidative Stress in PCOS

Conducting healthy lifestyle in women with PCOS did not demonstrate significant change in lipid levels. The effect of insulin-sensitizing drugs on dyslipidemia of PCOS is almost at the same level of efficacy as the lifestyle intervention. Metformin, the most investigated medication in PCOS in the recent time, has favorable effects on hyperinsulinemia, endothelium, restoration of ovulation, improving pregnancy rates and the number of live births. However, the effect of metformin as monotherapy on lipids in obese women with PCOS remains modest with mainly significant positive effect on the decrease in triglycerides. This effect disappears when metformin is used in combination with i.e. oral contraceptives [28]. Drugs from the thiazolidinedione class of insulin sensitizers like troglitazone or rosiglitazone did not show beneficial effects on deranged lipid profile in PCOS women even in a longer period of follow-up.

The tendency towards increasing the extent of plaque formation in the third decade of life suggests that risk factor modification in the population should be initiated almost in the second decade of life. When considering dyslipidemia as the most prevalent risk factor for cardiovascular disease overall, and in women with PCOS, there are no clear suggestions for the preventive or therapeutic use, or the age at which any HMG-CoA reductase inhibitor (statin) or other antilipemic drug for the treatment of dyslipidemia should be initiated. A recent Cochrane analysis of the studies with simvastatin and atorvastatin on the therapeutic outcomes in normal weight and obese women with PCOS showed that the use of statins was safe and effective in lowering testosterone levels, improving total cholesterol, LDL cholesterol

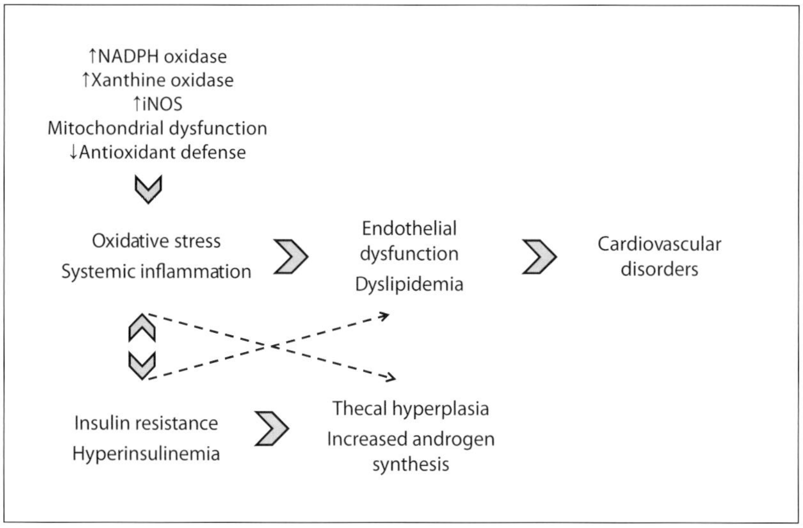

Fig. 1. Proposed role of oxidative stress and dyslipidemia in PCOS. Oxidative stress with systemic inflammation and insulin resistance promote dyslipidemia and endothelial dysfunction, as well as dysregulation of the ovarian thecal compartment.

and triglycerides but without significant effect on HDL cholesterol [29]. However, statins possess both indirect and direct antioxidant activity that includes inhibition of NADPH oxidase activity, preservation of relative levels of vitamins C and E, as well as inhibition of the uptake and generation of OxLDL. The intrinsic antioxidant activity of statins involves both anti-hydroxyl and anti-peroxyl radical activity. In vivo, statins reduce plasma levels of nitrotyrosine, and they also exert anti-inflammatory effects. Therefore, statins target not only dyslipidemia frequently associated with PCOS, but also the underlying stimulation of theca proliferation and steroidogenesis [27].

There is an established causative relation between PCOS and nonalcoholic fatty liver disease (NAFLD), conditions that are both associated with insulin resistance, obesity and MetSy. Supplementation with omega-3 fatty acids is considered to improve clinical features of NAFLD and have anti-inflammatory and antioxidant effect. Omega 3-fatty acids decrease liver fat content, triglycerides and blood pressure in obese women with PCOS, but it remains unanswered if these effects could be translated into reduction of cardiovascular morbidity [30].

Alpha lipoic acid is a potent antioxidant that improves insulin sensitivity and glucose control in patients with type 2 diabetes. However, in spite of beneficial effect on dyslipidemia in PCOS women, an antioxidant potential of α-lipoic acid has not been confirmed in these women yet. N-acetylcysteine is a thiol-containing antioxidant that elevates intracellular glutathione levels and increases insulin sensitivity in women with PCOS. These findings lead us towards evaluation of other antioxidants that could improve insulin sensitivity, increase ovulation rate, and reduce the risk for development of type 2 diabetes and cardiovascular disease in women with PCOS.

Conclusion

Dyslipidemia is certainly the most prevalent and persistent among cardiovascular risk factors in women with PCOS. This highly prevalent syndrome among women of reproductive age is considered as an insulin-resistant state closely related to the MetSy having a characteristic lipid profile with decreased HDL cholesterol and increased triglyceride levels. Oxidative stress has been established as a predisposing factor for the development of cardiovascular disease and a possible missing link towards pathological changes in a vulnerable endothelium. Recent studies showed an increased oxidative stress in women with PCOS that are prone to accumulate byproducts of lipid and protein oxidative damage in response to hyperglycemia and/or increased levels of free fatty acids. After years of looking for optimal therapeutic interventions in women of unstable metabolic state, as PCOS women are, today only statins seem to be a group of drugs that are effective and safe to ameliorate dyslipidemia and consequent oxidative stress. Another possibility for improvement of the proatherogenic profile lies among various supplements that are under broad investigation.

Acknowledgement

This work was supported by grants 41009 and 175052 from the Serbian Ministry of Science and Education.

References

1 Legro RS, Kunselman AR, Dunaif A: Prevalence and predictors of dyslipidemia in women with polycystic ovary syndrome. Am J Med 2001;111:607.

2 Gonzalez F, Rote NS, Minium J, Kirwan JP: Reactive oxygen species-induced oxidative stress in the development of insulin resistance and hyperandrogenism in polycystic ovary syndrome. J Clin Endocrinol Metab 2006;91:336.

3 Glintborg D, Mumm H, Hougaard D, Ravn P, Andersen M: Ethnic differences in rotterdam criteria and metabolic risk factors in a multiethnic group of women with PCOS studied in Denmark. Clin Endocrinol 2010;73:732.

4 Diamanti-Kandarakis E, Papavassiliou AG, Kandarakis SA, Chrousos GP: Pathophysiology and types of dyslipidemia in PCOS. Trends Endocrinol Metab 2007;18:280.

5 Hu Z, Wang Y, Qiao J, Li M, Chi H, Chen X: The role of family history in clinical symptoms and therapeutic outcomes of women with polycystic ovary syndrome. Int J Gynecol Obstet 2010;108:35.

6 Talbott E, Clerici A, Berga SL, Kuller L, Guzick D, Detre K, Daniels T, Engberg RA: Adverse lipid and coronary heart disease risk profiles in young women with polycystic ovary syndrome: results of a case-control study. J Clin Epidemiol 1998;51:415.

7 Macut D, Micić D, Cvijović G, Šumarac M, Kendereški A, Zorić S, Pejković D: Cardiovascular risk in adolescent and young adult obese females with polycystic ovary syndrome (PCOS). J Pediatr Endocrinol Metab 2001;14:1353.

8 Pirwany IR, Fleming R, Greer IA, Packard CJ, Sattar N: Lipids and lipoprotein subfractions in women with PCOS: relationship to metabolic and endocrine parameters. Clin Endocrinol (Oxf) 2001; 54:447.

9 Phelan N, O'Connor A, Kyaw-Tun T, Correia N, Boran G, Roche HM, Gibney J: Lipoprotein subclass patterns in women with polycystic ovary syndrome (PCOS) compared with equally insulin-resistant women without PCOS. J Clin Endocrinol Metab 2010;95:3933.

10 Macut D, Damjanović S, Panidis D, Spanos N, Glišić B, Petakov M, Rousso D, Kourtis A, Bjekić J, Milić N: Oxidised low-density lipoprotein concentration – early marker of an altered lipid metabolism in young women with PCOS. Eur J Endocrinol 2006; 155:131.
11 Berneis K, Rizzo M, Hersberger M, Rini GB, Di Fede G, Pepe I, Spinas GA, Carmina E: Atherogenic forms of dyslipidaemia in women with polycystic ovary syndrome. Int J Clin Pract 2009;63:56.
12 Koval KW, Setji TL, Reyes E, Brown AJ: Higher high-density lipoprotein cholesterol in African-American women with polycystic ovary syndrome compared with Caucasian counterparts. J Clin Endocrinol Metab 2010;95:E49.
13 Glueck CJ, Morrison JA, Goldenberg N, Wang P: Coronary heart disease risk factors in adult premenopausal white women. Metabolism 2009;58:714.
14 Wehr E, Grüber H-J, Giuliani A, Möller R, Pieber TR, Obermayer-Pietsch B: The lipid accumulation product is associated with impaired glucose tolerance in PCOS women. J Clin Endocrinol Metab 2011;96:E986.
15 Macut D, Panidis D, Glisić B, Spanos N, Petakov M, Bjekić J, Stanojlović O, Rousso D, Kourtis A, Bozić I, Damjanović S: Lipid and lipoprotein profile in women with polycystic ovary syndrome. Can J Physiol Pharmacol 2008;86:199.
16 Sies H: Oxidative stress: from basic research to clinical application. Am J Med 1991;91:31S.
17 Halliwell B: Reactive oxygen species in living systems. Source, biochemistry and role. Am J Med 1991;9:114.
18 Kuscu NK, Var A: Oxidative stress but not endothelial dysfunction exists in non-obese, young group of patients with polycystic ovary syndrome. Acta Obstet Gynecol 2009;88:612.
19 Macut D, Simic T, Lissounov A, Pljesa-Ercegovac M, Bozic I, Djukic T, Bjekic-Macut J, Matic M, Petakov M, Suvakov S, Damjanovic S, Savic-Radojevic A: Insulin resistance in non-obese women with polycystic ovary syndrome: relation to byproducts of oxidative stress. Exp Clin Endocrinol Diab 2011;119:451.
20 Fernández-Sánchez A, Madrigal-Santillán E, Bautista M, Esquivel-Soto J, Morales-González A, Esquivel-Chirino C, Durante-Montiel I, Sánchez-Rivera G, Valadez-Vega C, Morales-González JA: Inflammation, oxidative stress, and obesity. Int J Mol Sci 2011;12:3117.
21 Simic DV, Mimic-Oka J, Pljesa-Ercegovac M, Savic-Radojevic A, Opacic M, Matic D, Ivanovic B, Simic T: Byproducts of oxidative protein damage and antioxidant enzyme activities in plasma of patients with different degrees of essential hypertension. Hypertension 2006;20:149.
22 Victor M, Rocha M, Banuls C, Sanchez-Serrano M, Sola E, Gomez M, Hernandez-Mijares A: Mitochondrial complex I impairment in leukocytes from polycystic ovary syndrome patients with insulin resistance. J Clin Endocrinol Metab 2009;94: 3505.
23 Lee YS, Kim AY, Choi JW, Kim M, Yasue S, Son HJ, Masuzaki H, Park KS, Kim JB: Dysregulation of adipose glutathione peroxidase 3 in obesity contributes to local and systemic oxidative stress. Mol Endocrinol 2008;22:2176.
24 Yilmaz M, Bukan N, Ayvaz G, Karakoç A, Törüner F, Cakir N, Arslan M: The effects of rosiglitazone and metformin on oxidative stress and homocysteine levels in lean patients with polycystic ovary syndrome. Hum Reprod 2005;20:3333.
25 Evans J, Maddux BA, Goldfine ID: The molecular basis for oxidative stress-induced insulin resistance. Antioxid Redox Signal 2005;7:1040.
26 Duleba AJ, Foyouzi N, Karaca M, Pehlivan T, Kwintkiewicz J, Behrman HR: Proliferation of ovarian theca-interstitial cells is modulated by antioxidants and oxidative stress. Hum Reprod 2004;19: 1519.
27 Kodaman PH, Duleba AJ: Statins: do they have potential in the treatment of polycystic ovary syndrome? Semin Reprod Med 2008;26:127.
28 Hoeger K, Davidson K, Kochman L, Cherry T, Kopin L, Guzick DS: The impact of metformin, oral contraceptives, and lifestyle modification on polycystic ovary syndrome in obese adolescent women in two randomized, placebo-controlled clinical trials. J Clin Endocrinol Metab 2008;93:4299.
29 Raval AD, Hunter T, Stuckey B, Hart RJ: Statins for women with polycystic ovary syndrome not actively trying to conceive. Cochrane Database Syst Rev, DOI: 10.1002/14651858.
30 Cussons AJ, Watts GF, Mori TA, Stuckey BGA: Omega-3 fatty acid supplementation decreases liver fat content in polycystic ovary syndrome: a randomized controlled trial employing proton magnetic resonance spectroscopy. J Clin Endocrinol Metab 2009;94:3842.

Djuro Macut, MD, PhD
Clinic for Endocrinology, Diabetes and Metabolic Diseases
Faculty of Medicine, University of Belgrade
Dr Subotica 13
RS–11000 Belgrade (Serbia)
Tel. +381 11 3639744, E-Mail djmacut@gmail.com

Macut D, Pfeifer M, Yildiz BO, Diamanti-Kandarakis E (eds): Polycystic Ovary Syndrome. Novel Insights into Causes and Therapy. Front Horm Res. Basel, Karger, 2013, vol 40, pp 64–82

Cardiovascular Risk and Subclinical Cardiovascular Disease in Polycystic Ovary Syndrome

Katica Bajuk Studen · Mojca Jensterle Sever · Marija Pfeifer

Department of Endocrinology, Diabetes and Metabolic Diseases, University Medical Centre Ljubljana, Ljubljana, Slovenia

Abstract

In addition to its effects on reproductive health, it is now well recognized that polycystic ovary syndrome (PCOS) is a metabolic disorder, characterized by decreased insulin sensitivity which leads to an excess lifetime risk of type 2 diabetes and cardiovascular disease. PCOS patients are often obese, hypertensive, dyslipidemic and insulin resistant; they have obstructive sleep apnea and have been reported to have higher aldosterone levels in comparison to normal healthy controls. These are all components of an adverse cardiovascular risk profile. Many studies exploring subclinical atherosclerosis using different methods (flow-mediated dilatation, intima media thickness, arterial stiffness, coronary artery calcification) as well as assessing circulating cardiovascular risk markers, point toward an increased cardiovascular risk and early atherogenesis in PCOS. The risk and early features of subclinical atherosclerosis can be reversed by non-medical (normalization of weight, healthy life-style) and medical (metformin, thiazolidinediones, spironolactone, and statins) interventions. However, the long-term risk for cardiovascular morbidity and mortality as well as the clinical significance of different interventions still need to be properly addressed in a large prospective study.

Besides the clinical features of oligomenorrhea, hirsutism and infertility, polycystic ovary syndrome (PCOS) patients are often insulin resistant (IR), obese, they have arterial hypertension, dyslipidemia, an increased prothrombotic state, impaired glucose tolerance (IGT) or frank type 2 diabetes (T2D). High prevalence of cardiovascular risk factors in PCOS is assumed to be associated with accelerated cardiovascular disease (CVD). Since PCOS is highly prevalent in female population of the reproductive age accounting for 7–10% when applying National Institutes of Health 1990 criteria or even 15–20% by Rotterdam 2003 criteria, it represents a potential health

The first two authors should be regarded as joint first authors.

economic burden. However, clear data from large end point trials to answer the question about cardiovascular morbidity and mortality in PCOS are currently lacking. Of note, there are plenty of data on early occurrence of subclinical, potentially reversible atherosclerosis in women with PCOS, and many controlled clinical trials did show its amelioration with treatment and/or lifestyle changes.

Epidemiology of Cardiovascular Disease in PCOS

In one of the first studies addressing CVD, the association between polycystic ovaries (diagnosed by ultrasound only) and extent of coronary artery disease in 143 women having cardiac catheterization for assessment of chest pain or valvular disease was explored [1]. Polycystic ovaries were found in 42% of women, and those women had more extensive coronary artery disease than women with normal ovaries. The Nurses' Health Study included 82,439 female nurses who provided information in 1982 (at ages 20–35 years) on prior menstrual regularity and were followed through 1996 for cardiovascular events [2]. Incident reports of nonfatal myocardial infarction, fatal coronary heart disease (CHD), and nonfatal and fatal stroke were made. Compared with women reporting a history of very regular menstrual cycles, women reporting usually irregular or very irregular cycles (as a surrogate marker for PCOS) had an increased risk for nonfatal or fatal CHD.

Women's Ischemia Syndrome Evaluation study evaluated the risk of cardiovascular events in 390 postmenopausal women [3]. Hundred and four among them had clinical features of PCOS defined by a premenopausal history of irregular menses and current biochemical evidence of hyperandrogenemia. Women with clinical features of PCOS were more often diabetic, obese, with the metabolic syndrome and had more angiographic signs of coronary artery disease compared to women without clinical features of PCOS. Cumulative 5-year cardiovascular event-free survival was lower for women with clinical features of PCOS than for women without PCOS.

Three additional studies gave further support to the association between PCOS and CVD. The Rancho Bernardo cross-sectional study of 713 postmenopausal women (mean age, 73.8 years) showed that non-diabetic women with clinical and biochemical features of PCOS had significantly higher prevalence of CVD compared to women without that phenotype (RR 1.36, CI 1.05–1.76) [4]. A case-control study of 414 postmenopausal women (mean age, 60.4 years) reported an increased odds ratio for coronary vascular disease in women with premenopausal menstrual irregularity (as a putative sign of PCOS) [5]. In another study, increased waist/hip ratio and hirsutism were associated with confirmed coronary artery disease in women aged 60 years or older who underwent coronary angiography.

On the other hand, some studies have reported no association between the presence of PCOS and cardiovascular events. One of the population studies in the UK on 786 PCOS patients followed up for 30 years showed no increase in cardiovascular deaths compared to the national rate. A subsequent study by the same group found no difference in CHD morbidity and mortality between PCOS patients and age-matched controls [6]. Similarly, there was no difference in cardiac complaints between 346 PCOS patients and 8,950 controls, although the mean age of this cohort was only 39 years [7].

Even the most recent data are still contradictory. A large study (456,298.5 person-years of follow-up) reported an association between menstrual irregularity and increased age-adjusted risk for cardiovascular mortality [8]. However, this association was not statistically significant after adjustment for body mass index (BMI). These data are in conflict with another recent meta-analysis that showed a 2-fold risk for arterial disease in patients with PCOS as compared to women without PCOS [9]. BMI adjustment did not affect this finding.

The present epidemiological data suggest more frequent CVD in classical PCOS (as diagnosed by NIH criteria), mostly mediated through increased total and abdominal adiposity, and perhaps interacting with PCOS-related hyperandrogenism. In fact, both extremes of androgen levels in postmenopausal women, in either direction, are associated with increased risk of CVD. Several studies have indicated that low levels of testosterone are associated with more carotid atherosclerosis compared to higher, but normal levels of testosterone [10]. On the other hand, in the Multi-Ethnic Study of Atherosclerosis, 1,947 women were evaluated for subclinical atherosclerosis according to their circulating androgens. Testosterone levels correlated positively with carotid intima media thickness, independently of BMI and IR [11]. In the analysis of the Rancho Bernardo population, women in the highest quintile of circulating testosterone had an increased incidence of CVD over 20 years of follow-up (RR 1.96, CI 1.13–3.41) compared to women in the middle quintile, independent of age, BMI, smoking and central adiposity [4]. However, according to several other trials, the contribution of coexisting risk factors to CVD in women with higher androgen levels should always be taken into account.

In conclusion, women with PCOS often have an adverse cardiovascular risk profile. However, data on long-term risk for cardiovascular morbidity and mortality are inconsistent, and this issue has not been properly addressed by a large prospective study yet.

Cardiovascular Risk Factors in PCOS

Data on CVD and cardiovascular mortality in women with PCOS are thus insufficient. This paucity of data is, in part, due to the fact that most studies in this population are conducted at a time when women are young, before an age when CVD would be expected to develop. Due to the lack of outcome studies, a wealth of traditional as well as less traditional surrogate risk markers is very important and points toward an increased cardiovascular risk in women with PCOS.

It has long been established that obesity, particularly of visceral origin, plays a crucial role in both the development and maintenance of PCOS, and significantly influences the severity of cardiovascular risk profile. In most large series, at least 30% of women with PCOS are obese, and in some series, up to 75% are obese. About 50–60% of women with PCOS have central body fat distribution whereby a disproportionate quantity of adipose tissue is distributed in the visceral depot. Visceral fat is the main source of free fatty acids and inflammatory cytokines causing IR and consequent CVD. Furthermore, mean arterial blood pressure and the risk of preeclampsia are higher in women with PCOS. Lipid abnormalities are encountered in up to 70% of PCOS patients.

Beyond the traditional CVD risk factors, more recently identified risk markers are also more prevalent in women with PCOS. In a recent meta-analysis looking into the relationship between PCOS and CVD, various risk markers were analyzed [12]. Women with PCOS had significantly elevated high-sensitivity C-reactive protein (hsCRP), homocysteine, plasminogen activator inhibitor-1 and its activity, vascular endothelial growth factor, asymmetric dimethylarginine, advanced glycation end products (AGEs), and lipoprotein(a) concentrations compared with controls, yet with significant between-study heterogeneity [12].

AGEs have been shown to be increased in PCOS women, independent of obesity and insulin resistance. In postmenopausal women, higher levels of AGEs were positively associated with higher androgen levels suggesting a potential pathophysiological mechanism contributing to higher prevalence of cardiovascular events in postmenopausal women with higher androgen levels. Endothelin-1, a marker of abnormal vascular reactivity, was also increased in women with PCOS compared with the age-matched controls, independently of the presence of obesity. A positive correlation of endothelin-1 with free testosterone levels and a negative correlation with insulin sensitivity were also observed.

Insulin Resistance in PCOS

IR is highly prevalent, occurring in 60–80% of women with PCOS and in 95% of obese women with PCOS. It is most prevalent and severe in classic PCOS phenotype with hyperandrogenism and chronic anovulation. IR is intrinsic to the disorder and additive with that of obesity. PCOS and obesity act synergistically to impair insulin sensitivity. In vivo insulin action is profoundly decreased in skeletal muscle secondary to signaling defects, but hepatic IR is present only in obese women with PCOS. There is a defect in insulin postreceptor signaling, namely increased serin/threonin phosphorylation of insulin receptor substrates (IRSs) instead of tyrosine phosphorylation, and consequent proteosomic degradation of IRSs.

IR plays a central pathogenetic role in the development of metabolic derangements of the syndrome like IGT, T2D, atherogenic dyslipidemia, chronic inflammation and others. IGT and T2D are highly prevalent among PCOS adolescents, and up to 40% of women with classic PCOS develop IGT or T2D by the fourth decade of life, with age and weight gain worsening the glycemic control [13].

In the arterial wall, IR is associated with reduced synthesis and release of nitric oxide (NO), enhanced inactivation of NO after its release from endothelial cells and enhanced synthesis of vasoconstricting agents. Increased vascular stiffness and impaired vasodilatory action of insulin ex vivo was demonstrated in patients with PCOS suggesting an abnormal insulin-regulated endothelial NO production in the vasculature [14]. In addition, it has been demonstrated that hyperinsulinemia exerts a direct hypertrophic effect on the vascular endothelium and the smooth muscle cells. In the arteries of skeletal muscles, insulin can stimulate both endothelin-1 and NO production, and an imbalance between the release of these two substances may be involved in the pathophysiology of endothelial dysfunction. More accurately, phosphatidylinositol 3 kinase (PI3 kinase)-dependent insulin-signaling pathway which stimulates NO production in the endothelium shares striking similarities with the metabolic pathway in the skeletal muscle that promotes glucose uptake. Other distinct nonmetabolic pathway of insulin-signaling (mitogen-activated protein kinase, MAP kinase, pathway) stimulates secretion of the vasoconstrictor endothelin-1 in the endothelium. IR is characterized by pathway-specific impairment in PI3 kinase-dependent signaling, leaving MAP kinase pathway unaffected, which in endothelium may cause imbalance between production of NO and secretion of endothelin-1. Increased endothelin-1 levels have already been demonstrated in PCOS population [15].

It has also been suggested that inflammatory markers such as hsCRP directly promote the atherosclerotic processes and endothelial cell inflammation leading to atherothrombosis. Furthermore, IR is linked to the endothelial dysfunction also by other mechanisms, such as increased oxidative stress, increased activity of the renin-angiotensin system and the action of hormones and cytokines secreted by the adipose tissue.

Arterial Hypertension

Hypertension is a significant contributor to the risk of CVD. Although hypertension has been an inconsistent finding, several studies suggest its increased prevalence in women with PCOS compared with the general population. The prevalence of hypertension in PCOS ranges from 10 to 40% [16]. In addition, there are some data to suggest that the nocturnal decrease in blood pressure characteristic of healthy vasculature is absent in adolescent and adult women with PCOS and that pregnant women with PCOS have a greater risk of pregnancy-induced hypertension and preeclampsia than pregnant women without PCOS. Obesity may have a major influence on blood pressure in PCOS. In the studies that did adjust the analyses for BMI, the association between hypertension and PCOS was not always clear. However, there are several other mechanisms potentially involved in the pathogenesis of hypertension in PCOS. Increased blood pressure may be secondary to enhanced sodium retention occurring in the setting of IR. Hyperandrogenemia has been associated with hypertension in

PCOS independent of obesity and hyperinsulinemia. Greater sympathetic activity has also been implicated in the etiology of hypertension in this population.

Given the association of hypertension with all of the common PCOS manifestations, treating the manifestations of PCOS may treat concomitant hypertension or the risk for hypertension as well. Lifestyle modifications and other methods of weight loss were shown to improve hypertension. The response to oral contraceptives has been inconsistent. There are data to suggest that the effect of spironolactone is beneficial [17]. Antihypertensives are indicated for blood pressure of at least 140 mm Hg systolic or 90 mm Hg diastolic. Reducing blood pressure to 120/80 mm Hg is optimal for long-term CVD prevention. Some authors favor angiotensin-converting enzyme inhibitors and angiotensin receptor blockers over diuretics and beta-blockers. It would be prudent to avoid using agents that impair insulin sensitivity (atenolol, metoprolol). All above-mentioned antihypertensives are contraindicated in pregnancy and require contraception.

The Androgen Excess and Polycystic Ovarian Disease Society recommends a screening blood pressure measurement in women with PCOS at every visit and that prehypertension and hypertension are detected and treated, given the potential benefit of lowering blood pressure for the prevention of CVD [13].

Dyslipidemia

PCOS is frequently, but not always, associated with dyslipidemia. Dyslipidemia in PCOS can present with different patterns: lower levels of high-density lipoprotein cholesterol (HDL cholesterol) and higher levels of triglycerides, total and low-density lipoprotein cholesterol (LDL cholesterol) [18]. Different types of dyslipidemia are probably the net result of interfering influences of hyperandrogenism, IR and additional environmental influences (diet, exercise) and genetics. Obese PCOS patients most frequently have the so-called atherogenic type of dyslipidemia with low HDL cholesterol, small dense LDL particles and elevated triglyceride levels, which is typical for states with IR. Because the pathophysiologic processes of obesity and IR overlap, this form of dyslipidemia most often presents in obese PCOS patients (which represent 70% of the PCOS population in the USA). However, in countries with lower average BMI, this association is less frequent [18]. A form of dyslipidemia with high LDL cholesterol was reported in PCOS, but is less frequent, less obesity correlated and more hyperandrogenism correlated [19; see the chapter on dyslipidemia and oxidative stress by Macut et al., pp. 51–63].

The Renin-Angiotensin-Aldosterone System in PCOS

Many experimental and clinical data show that aldosterone is an important risk factor for CVD [20]. Aldosterone accelerates fibrosis in the myocardium and blood vessels, negatively affects the compliance of arteries, remodeling of the heart muscle and causes perivascular inflammation. The main etiopathogenetic event behind these cardiovascular changes could be an immunostimulatory state, characterized by oxidative stress, inflammation and profibrogenic genotype. Data on association of aldosterone with IGT, T2D and metabolic syndrome are also accumulating. Even values of aldosterone in the upper normal range are associated with arterial hypertension, although the deleterious effects of aldosterone on cardiovascular system are independent of its effects on blood pressure.

One of the first papers studying the renin-angiotensin-aldosterone system in PCOS reported higher levels of renin in PCOS patients compared to the control group, which was explained by greater activity of intrinsic renin-angiotensin-aldosterone system in ovaria. Other studies also reported higher levels of angiotensin II, although not all the data are consistent.

In a later report that included 50 PCOS patients and 50 healthy controls, plasma concentration of aldosterone in association with cardiovascular risk factors was studied [21]. Aldosterone but not renin levels were significantly increased in the PCOS group. In PCOS, a significant direct correlation between plasma aldosterone and fasting insulin concentration, homeostasis model assessment index of IR (HOMAIR), hsCRP, intima media thickness (IMT), and mean blood pressure was found. This was later confirmed by other studies.

Regarding the renin-angiotensin-aldosterone system, the question of medical intervention arises. Namely, low-dose spironolactone (an antimineralocorticoid and antiandrogenic drug) treatment without any relevant hemodynamic effect significantly improved survival and endothelial function in patients with chronic heart failure. This finding revolutionized the treatment of heart failure several years ago. Since spironolactone is routinely used for treating hyperandrogenism in PCOS patients, it could have additional beneficial effect in lowering cardiovascular risk. Our group was the first to report that it improved endothelial dysfunction in non-obese, non-insulin-resistant PCOS patients [22]. However, it was also shown that spironolactone worsened endothelial function in type 2 diabetic patients, probably due to worsening of glycemic control and an increase in angiotensin II [23]. Since many of the PCOS patients have IGT or T2D, they most probably represent a subgroup in which the beneficial effect of spironolactone is less likely. Before firmer instructions on therapy can be stated, further research in this area is needed.

Obstructive Sleep Apnea in PCOS Women

Adult (but not adolescent) PCOS patients were reported to have at least 5-fold higher risk for obstructive sleep apnea (OSA) as similarly obese women without PCOS. OSA is an independent risk factor for CVD. It is associated with activated pathways that lead to IR, hypertension and increased levels of a group of proinflammatory and prothrombotic factors that are involved in the atherogenetic process. Therefore, OSA may be an underrecognized yet significant risk factor for cardiometabolic derangements in PCOS which can be successfully treated [24]. In an 8-week study on 56 PCOS patients, 26 among them having OSA, insulin sensitivity parameters improved, sympathetic tone decreased and diastolic blood pressure reduced after treatment with continuous positive airway pressure [25].

The association between hormonal derangements in PCOS and development of OSA has not been thoroughly studied yet. Several studies have reported a protective role of estrogens and progestins against the development of OSA in women, among them a study by Polo-Kantola's group which showed a small yet clinically significant decrease in the occurrence and frequency of sleep apnea in postmenopausal women receiving estrogen replacement rather than placebo. High levels of progesterone in the luteal phase of the menstrual cycle are thought to be associated with lower upper airway resistance and direct stimulation of the respiratory drive by increased ventilatory response to both hypercapnia and hypoxemia and therefore protective against OSA. However, the oligo-/anovulation state often seen in PCOS women is associated with lower progesterone levels, and this may be an important cause of the higher prevalence of OSA in PCOS. Testosterone was reported to influence both neural control of breathing and upper airway mechanics. In a small study on premenopausal women treated with testosterone, Zhou and colleagues reported increased apneic threshold suggesting increased breathing instability during sleep in that cohort. Several studies performed by Shinohara and Hoffstein's groups have shown a correlation of the OSA risk with the total body fat mass as well as body fat distribution. This may be important for PCOS women who typically have increased abdominal fat which highly correlates with increased OSA risk.

Subclinical Cardiovascular Disease in PCOS

It has been established in many studies that beyond CVD risk factors, PCOS patients have earlier subclinical CVD compared with age- and BMI-matched controls.

Methods Evaluating Subclinical Atherosclerosis

There are various invasive (coronary angiography, intravascular ultrasound) and, more commonly used, noninvasive methods to evaluate atherosclerosis even at a subclinical stage when patients are still asymptomatic. With these techniques, different parameters of the atherosclerotic process such as endothelial dysfunction, vessel wall thickness, luminal diameter or stenosis, plaque volume, and the specific distribution and localization of atherosclerotic disease can be validated.

Flow-Mediated Dilation of the Brachial Artery

This method evaluates endothelial function by measuring flow-mediated dilation (FMD) of the brachial artery in response to shear stress using ultrasound. Increased shear stress (caused by increased blood flow to the transitory ischemic distal arm, after releasing the inflated sphygmomanometer cuff) induces endothelium-dependent dilation of the artery, mainly mediated by NO. FMD is usually reported as percentage change from the baseline diameter of the brachial artery. FMD correlates significantly with coronary endothelial function and with the extent and severity of coronary atherosclerosis.

Intima-Media Thickness

The combined thickness of the arterial intimal and medial layers (usually in the common carotid artery) can be measured by using B-mode ultrasonography. The carotid IMT reflects the diffuse thickening of the intimal layer seen in atherosclerosis and has been validated as a measure of the risk for cardiovascular events and atherosclerotic disease burden.

Pulse Wave Velocity

Pulse wave velocity (PWV) is a measure of arterial stiffness. It can be measured invasively and noninvasively in humans; it is highly reproducible, and there is a strong correlation between PWV and future cardiovascular events.

Electron-Beam Computed Tomography

Electron-beam computed tomography (EBCT) is used in clinical practice and measures coronary artery calcification (CAC) reflecting plaque burden, as calcium deposits are related to the lipid and apoptotic remnants of the plaque. CAC is an independent cardiovascular risk factor. However, although EBCT can localize coronary plaques within the coronary tree and provide a quantitative measure of relative disease severity, it cannot be used to ascertain the susceptibility of individual plaques to rupture.

High-Resolution MRI

MRI non-invasively evaluates plaque volume and composition, fibrous cap integrity, and lesion type. Consequently, it provides a measure of both plaque burden and susceptibility to rupture.

We need to stress that some of the above-described methods are currently used only in clinical trial settings and are not yet developed enough for individual patient management.

Endothelial Dysfunction

Vascular endothelium has an important role in maintaining vascular homeostasis by influencing vascular tone, cell adhesion, smooth muscle cell proliferation, inflammation in the vascular wall and resistance to thrombosis in response to various chemical and physical signals [26]. Many of those functions are regulated by NO bio-availability. NO is produced in vascular endothelium from L-arginine by the constitutive NO synthase.

NO is a key signaling molecule for maintaining vascular wall in quiescent state by inhibiting inflammation, cell proliferation and thrombosis. This effect is mediated by S-nitrosylation of cysteine residues of many proteins (for example transcription factor NFκB, proteins of the cell cycle, etc.) reducing their biological activity. NO also inhibits oxidative phosphorylation in mitochondria and consequent generation of reactive oxygen species (ROS).

Specific circumstances lead to endothelium activation, which is characterized by a 'switch' of endothelial NO synthase, which instead of NO generates ROS. ROS generate hydrogen peroxide, which is like NO capable of fast diffusion. It interacts with cysteine residues of proteins and thereby affects their function. However, due to different biochemical processes this leads to phosphorylation of transcription factors, remodeling of the nuclear chromatin and activation of proteases.

Activation of the endothelium is sometimes part of a normal defense of the host to the invasion of microorganisms. In such circumstances, a coordinated function of chemokines, cytokines and adhesion molecules is needed to provide efficient interaction with leukocytes. This adaptation mechanism of endothelium can become proatherogenic under pathologic circumstances, for example hyperlipidemia, arterial hypertension, IR and also other conditions, associated with chronic inflammation (periodontitis). Under such circumstances chronic production of ROS overrides the capacity of cellular enzyme and non-enzyme antioxidants, and this can through continuous activation of endothelium lead to vascular disease.

It is known now that these early changes in endothelial function precede morphologic changes. In later stages of atherosclerosis, changes in endothelial function lead to the inflammation process in the atherosclerotic artery, which can destabilize the atherosclerotic plaque and promote clinical events such as myocardial infarction.

To sum up, endothelial dysfunction represents an early, preclinical state of the atherosclerotic process, which is potentially reversible. The measurement of endothelial function represents an important tool to study future morbidity from atherosclerotic disease as well as to study the effect of different interventions to prevent CVD. Several mechanisms may be involved in the development of endothelial dysfunction in PCOS, IR probably playing the key role among them.

Endothelial dysfunction contributes to CVDs (hypertension, coronary artery disease, peripheral arterial disease), which are also characterized by IR [27]. On the other hand, IR is a cornerstone of metabolic disorders, including PCOS, obesity and T2D mellitus, which are also characterized by endothelial dysfunction. Glucose disposal is promoted by metabolic actions of insulin, but is also augmented by vascular actions of insulin in endothelium stimulating production of NO. It was shown that NO-dependent increases in blood flow to skeletal muscle account for 25–40% of the

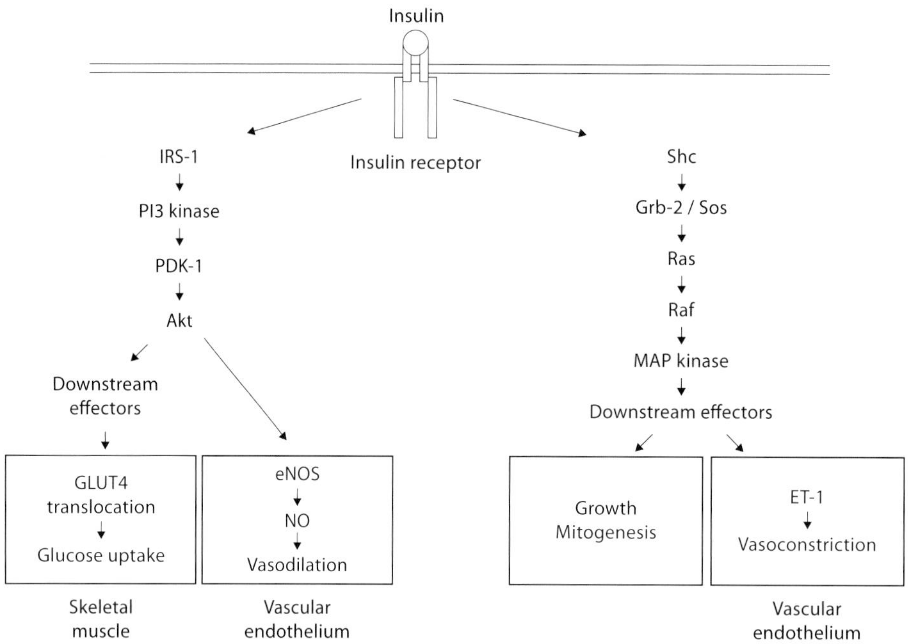

Fig. 1. General features of insulin signal transduction pathways. PI3 kinase pathway of insulin signaling regulates GLUT4 translocation and glucose uptake in skeletal muscle and NO production and vasodilation in vascular endothelium. MAP kinase pathway of insulin signaling generally regulates growth and mitogenesis and controls secretion of ET-1 in vascular endothelium. Reprinted with permission from Kim et al. [27].

increase in glucose uptake in response to insulin stimulation. Insulin-signaling pathways in endothelium which are related to production of NO and are mediated by PI3 kinase have many similarities with metabolic pathways in skeletal muscle that promote glucose uptake. Furthermore, secretion of the vasoconstrictor endothelin-1 in endothelium is regulated by other distinct nonmetabolic MAP kinase pathways of insulin signaling. Metabolic IR is characterized by pathway-specific impairment in PI3 kinase-dependent signaling, which in endothelium may cause imbalance between production of NO and secretion of endothelin-1, leading to vasoconstriction and decreased blood flow, which worsens IR (fig. 1). Different therapeutic interventions have shown that improving endothelial function ameliorates IR, whereas improving insulin sensitivity ameliorates endothelial function. Based on different basic and clinical studies, we can conclude that there is a tight relationship between endothelial dysfunction and IR that links cardiovascular and metabolic diseases.

Endothelial dysfunction in PCOS patients was first described by Paradisi et al. [28] in 2001. They studied 12 obese PCOS patients and 13 age- and weight-matched controls by invasively measuring blood flow responses to graded intrafemoral artery infusions of the endothelium-dependent vasodilator metacholine chloride. Leg blood flow increments in response to metacholine were significantly lower in the PCOS group than in the controls. They also showed that endothelial dysfunction in PCOS was associated with higher levels of androgens and with IR. Their findings were confirmed by many, although not all later studies, using different methods of assessing endothelial function. Women with PCOS have significant endothelial dysfunction already at an early age (i.e. in early 20s), and it is largely independent of obesity. A trend of deterioration of endothelial function from lean to overweight and obese PCOS women was observed in one study, but differences among groups were not statistically significant [29].

Intima Media Thickness

The pathological changes in the arterial vessel wall develop during a long subclinical lag phase in the atherogenetic process. This subclinical phase is characterized by gradual thickening of the intima. Therefore, the measurement of the IMT of large superficial arteries, especially the carotid artery, has emerged as one of the methods for evaluating the extent of damage to the arterial wall and for assessing cardiovascular risk, with good reproducibility. IMT has been shown to be associated with the extent of atherosclerosis and end-organ damage of high-risk patients. Both the carotid and femoral IMTs increase significantly with age, cholesterol level and hypertension. IMT was shown to be greater in men than in women and is affected by adverse lifestyle factors (cholesterol intake, BMI, and smoking). Increased IMT is correlated with angiographically assessed coronary artery disease and the extent of CAC, peripheral arterial occlusive disease and the prevalence of abdominal aortic aneurysm.

Increased IMT reflects the atherosclerotic burden and is a good predictor of subsequent events. Because of its quantitative value, carotid IMT is frequently used in clinical trials to test the effect of different preventive measures, including drugs, and could be used in the future for identifying subjects at high risk. Guzick and colleagues evaluated 16 hyperandrogenic premenopausal women at least 40 years of age, diagnosed previously with PCOS, compared with 16 age-matched regularly cycling controls undergoing carotid artery scanning, and found mean carotid IMT significantly greater in PCOS patients (0.68 mm) than controls (0.63 mm). However, the mean IMT in the PCOS group was still well below that seen in patients with significant carotid artery disease. Talbott's group evaluated 125 Caucasian women with PCOS and 142 age-matched controls, and confirmed greater carotid IMT in PCOS patients (0.78 mm) than controls 45 years of age and older (0.70 mm), which remained significant after adjusting for BMI. There was no difference between IMT in PCOS and controls in the group aged 30–44 years. These results suggest that lifelong exposure to an adverse cardiovascular risk profile in PCOS may lead to premature atherosclerosis and that PCOS-IMT association is explained only in part by weight and fat distribution and associated risk factors. There may be an independent effect of PCOS per se unexplained by the above variables that is related to hormonal dysregulation in this condition.

Several further studies confirmed the increased IMT in PCOS patients in comparison to healthy controls, among them a study by Lakhani and colleagues in 2004 and by Orio and colleagues in 2004, who showed increased IMT in young, normal-weight, nondyslipidemic, nonhypertensive women with PCOS.

The effect of intervention with metformin on IMT in PCOS was also studied, with discordant results. Orio's group showed reversal of IMT after 6 months of treatment with metformin 850 mg daily. However, in a study published by Sahin and colleagues, PCOS subjects were treated for 6 months with metformin 2,550 mg/day without a remarkable effect on IMT.

Arterial Stiffness

In the pathogenesis of atherosclerosis, vascular calcification is an active and complex process that involves numerous mechanisms responsible for calcium depositions in arterial walls, as described by Karwowsky and colleagues in 2012. They lead to an increase in arterial stiffness and in PWV, which in turn increases CVD morbidity and mortality. Calcification of vessels reduces their elasticity, affecting hemodynamic parameters of the cardiovascular system and leading to arterial hypertension, cardiac hypertrophy, ischemic heart disease or peripheral arterial disease in later stages. The extent of accumulation of calcium deposits in vessel walls is a key risk factor of ischemic events. Therefore understanding of vascular calcification mechanisms may be crucial for establishing an effective vasculoprotective therapy in the earlier stages of the disease.

Increased PWV in PCOS was first demonstrated by Kelly et al. [14] in 2002. Their findings suggested IR at a vascular level in women without overt CVD. This was later confirmed by Meyer's group in 2005 and several other studies, but not Cussons' study in 2009.

A study published in 2010 by Agarwal and colleagues explored the effect of metformin treatment (500 mg 3 times daily, 12 weeks) on arterial stiffness. They found an improvement in large artery stiffness with metformin therapy as evidenced by a reduction in an augmentation index and slowed brachial and aortic PWV. In contrast to these results, Meyer and colleagues in 2007 failed to detect a change in PWV with 6 months of metformin treatment in their population of women with PCOS, but did note an increase in PWV with a high-dose oral contraceptive (35 μg ethinyl estradiol/2 mg cyproterone acetate). These divergent effects on arterial stiffness of the two most commonly prescribed treatments for young women with PCOS could thus have important practical implications for considering choice of therapy in the clinic. However, in contrast to the findings of Agarwals' group, the participants in Meyer's study did not lose weight; neither did their blood pressure change, which suggests that the vascular improvements observed with metformin might be dependent at least in part on changes in these variables.

Coronary Artery Calcification

A study published by Christian and colleagues in 2003 explored the prevalence and predictors of CAC in women with PCOS, using EBCT. PCOS women, especially the obese cohort, were found to have greater prevalence and extent of CAC than unaffected women. These results were later confirmed by Talbott and colleagues in 2004. Using National Institutes of Health criteria and adjusting for age and BMI, both studies suggest that women with PCOS have a greater CAC prevalence than controls, independent of age and BMI, although small sample sizes and the young age of the population precluded analysis of a range of CAC.

Medical Interventions and Cardiovascular Risk in PCOS

Lifestyle Changes

Lifestyle modification is regarded as the first-line treatment for women with PCOS for the avoidance of CVD. It has been shown that even modest short-term weight loss of less than 10% decreases abdominal fat and improves insulin sensitivity, hyperglycemia, androgenicity, depression, frequency of ovulation, conception and quality of life. Up to 60% of PCOS women had improvement in either menstrual cycle or ovulation after lifestyle changes and subsequent weight loss [30]. In one study, both IR and visceral fat decreased significantly after 12 weeks of intensive supervised exercise. Since exercise and weight loss also improve dyslipidemia, lifestyle modification is particularly important for those individuals with serum LDL cholesterol levels >160 mg/dl (4 mmol/l) and/or non-HDL cholesterol levels at least 190 mg/dl (5 mmol/l) [31].

The Androgen Excess and Polycystic Ovarian Syndrome Society recommends a hypocaloric, low saturated fat, increased mono- and polyunsaturated fat diet (500–1,000 kcal/day reduction; <30% calories from fat, <10% calories from saturated fat, increased consumption of fiber, whole grain breads, cereals, fruits and vegetables), along with at least 30 min of moderate intensity physical activity daily. Overweight/obese PCOS women should initially attempt 5–10% weight loss to reduce obesity-related CVD risk factors, with long-term goals of achieving and maintaining reduced weight of 10–20% and a waist circumference of <80–88 cm, depending upon ethnicity [13]. Modifying dietary macronutrient composition does not seem to offer benefit for weight loss over conventional dietary approaches alone.

One of the main challenges of lifestyle changes is the low participants' compliance rate over time. Therefore, pharmaceutical intervention is an additional therapeutic tool to lifestyle changes in many patients.

Medical Therapy

Metformin
Metformin is the most extensively studied insulin-sensitizing agent for the treatment of women with PCOS. Its primary action is on the liver, where it increases insulin sensitivity and inhibits hepatic glucose production. Extrahepatic sites of action include the skeletal muscles, adipose tissue, endothelium, and the ovary. It enhances peripheral tissue sensitivity to insulin, necessitating a lower insulin concentration and thereby probably reducing the androgen production of theca cells in ovaries. The actual protection of metformin from cardiovascular morbidity and mortality has yet to be demonstrated. There is some evidence of beneficial activity on surrogate cardiovascular risk markers. It may improve atherogenic dyslipidemia, increasing HDL cholesterol and decreasing triglycerides, although the results are inconsistent. It does not improve LDL cholesterol or non-HDL-cholesterol, and should not be used alone when these lipid parameters are elevated [32]. There are inconclusive results regarding its effect on endothelial function in PCOS. Its administration has been proven beneficial in few studies: endothelial dysfunction was reversed to control levels in 20 PCOS patients [32] and improved in 30 nondyslipidemic, nonhypertensive, young, normal-weight women with PCOS, 6 months after metformin treatment [33]. On the other hand, endothelial dysfunction did not improve after 6 months of metformin treatment in a larger controlled trial published by Meyer and colleagues in 2007.

Thiazolidinediones
Currently, there are limited data on the use of thiazolidinediones (TZDs) in PCOS. TZDs exert their insulin-sensitizing actions through the peroxisome proliferator-activated receptor (PPAR)-γ found in a number of tissues including the liver, the skeletal muscle, and the adipose tissue. Troglitazone, which is now unavailable, due to hepatic toxicity, is the most researched agent in PCOS. It produced significant endocrine, metabolic and ovulatory benefits [34]. Rosiglitazone, the representative of a new generation of TZDs, has been shown to increase ovulation rates, reduce hyperandrogenism and improve the metabolic profile. There are more limited data on the beneficial effects of rosiglitazone on the endothelial function. Rosiglitazone was shown to improve endothelial dysfunction in non-obese young women with PCOS, where a significant association between beneficial effect on endothelial function and an improvement in insulin sensitivity was also reported [35]. In the study by our group, we demonstrated that both metformin and rosiglitazone administration significantly improved FMD of the brachial artery in young women with PCOS, metformin being as effective as rosiglitazone. We followed young PCOS patients without any clinical signs of atherosclerosis who were not severely IR (as assessed by HOMAIR), which enabled us to demonstrate that therapeutic interventions with insulin sensitizers may reverse the atherosclerotic process in young women at its early stage [36]. However, regarding translation of these data to clinical use in PCOS, it

needs to be acknowledged, that because of an uncertain safety profile in pregnancy, rosiglitazone should not be prescribed to women wishing to conceive. Furthermore, increased fracture risk and exacerbation of preexisting congestive heart failure, a significant increase in the risk of myocardial infarction in patients with T2D mellitus, limit TZDs use for primary CVD prevention in PCOS population. In addition, TZDs cause weight gain that is absolutely not a desirable effect in this population. Therefore, most investigators favor metformin over TZDs in PCOS treatment.

Drospirenone

Many patients with PCOS are treated with oral contraceptive agents (OCPs) for their menstrual irregularity and hirsutism. Drospirenone (DRSP) is a 17α spironolactone derivative progestin that combines progestogenic with antiandrogenic and antimineralocorticoid activity. The results of trials of its potentially beneficial cardiovascular risk profile are inconclusive. In a study of 16 lean and 12 overweight PCOS subjects, 6 months of 30 μg ethinyl estradiol and 3 mg of DRSP (EE/DRSP) treatment showed no effects on endothelial function or cardiovascular risk indices [37].

A study of EE/DRSP showed an increase in systolic, diastolic and 24-hour blood pressure of about 5 mm Hg and an increase in triglyceride levels. Another study demonstrated a more convincing decrease in systolic blood pressure in response to DRSP-containing combined OCP compared with a small increase in systolic blood pressure in the desogestrel-containing combined OCP group of women with PCOS. However, some investigations in PCOS demonstrated no change in blood pressure with an EE/DRSP. The optimal estrogen-containing OCP for PCOS needs clarification, but these studies suggest that the combination of 20 μg ethinyl estradiol with 3 mg DRSP may at least be neutral on cardiovascular risk [38].

Incretin Mimetics Therapy

An altered secretion pattern and/or insulinotropic activity of glucagon-like peptide-1 (GLP-1) have been described in diabetes and in other conditions connected with impaired glucose regulation. Although progressive IR plays a key role in the predisposition to diabetes in PCOS, subtle alterations in insulin secretion related to insulinotropic activity of GLP-1 also appear to contribute to the susceptibility toward T2D [39]. Therapy with GLP-1 agonists often results in weight loss, which further assists in decreasing IR. To date, there is only one 24-week randomized controlled trial in women with PCOS using GLP-1 mimetics. A combination treatment with exenatide (GLP-1 mimetic) and metformin was found to be superior to exenatide or metformin monotherapy in reducing weight (mean weight loss of 6 ± 0.5 kg) and improving menstrual cycles, ovulation rate, free androgen index, and insulin sensitivity [40]. Most commonly reported side effects are nausea and vomiting, but the main safety concern is a possible increased risk of pancreatitis which is attributable to drugs that act through the GLP-1 pathway. One of the disadvantages of using GLP-1R agonists is that they require injection. Although not yet licensed for obesity management,

GLP-1R agonists offer a potential obesity treatment and CVD protection for women with PCOS.

Conclusion

In this chapter, we focused on different cardiovascular risk factors that are more prevalent in PCOS patients than in the normal healthy population. Although the definitive risk for increased cardiovascular morbidity and mortality of PCOS patients still needs to be evidence based, many studies are strongly suggestive of this. Different methods of evaluating subclinical atherosclerosis indicate accelerated atherogenesis in PCOS that can be reversed by various medical and lifestyle interventions. Based on the available data, we conclude that besides the management of their reproductive and cosmetic issues, PCOS patients also need a thorough workup of their metabolic and cardiovascular risk factors, implementing lifestyle management as primary CVD prevention and adding insulin-sensitizing and other drugs if dyslipidemia or other risk factors persist.

References

1 Birdsall MA, Farquhar CM, White HD: Association between polycystic ovaries and extent of coronary artery disease in women having cardiac catheterization. Ann Intern Med 1997;126:32.

2 Solomon CG, Hu FB, Dunaif A, Rich-Edwards JE, Stampfer MJ, Willett WC, Speizer FE, Manson JE: Menstrual cycle irregularity and risk for future cardiovascular disease. J Clin Endocrinol Metab 2002; 87:2013.

3 Shaw LJ, Bairey Merz CN, Azziz R, et al: Postmenopausal women with a history of irregular menses and elevated androgen measurements at high risk for worsening cardiovascular event-free survival: results from the National Institutes of Health–National Heart, Lung, and Blood Institute Sponsored Women's Ischemia Syndrome Evaluation. J Clin Endocrinol Metab 2008;93:1276.

4 Krentz AJ, von Mühlen D, Barrett-Connor E: Searching for polycystic ovary syndrome in postmenopausal women: evidence of a dose-effect association with prevalent cardiovascular disease. Menopause 2007;14:284.

5 Azevedo GD, Duarte JM, Souza MO, Costa-E-Silva TD, Soares EM, Maranhão TM: Menstrual cycle irregularity as a marker of cardiovascular risk factors at postmenopausal years. Arq Bras Endocrinol Metabol 2006;50:876.

6 Wild S, Pierpoint T, McKeigue P, Jacobs H: Cardiovascular disease in women with polycystic ovary syndrome at long-term follow-up: a retrospective cohort study. Clin Endocrinol (Oxf) 2000; 52:595.

7 Elting MW, Korsen TJ, Bezemer PD, Schoemaker J: Prevalence of diabetes mellitus, hypertension and cardiac complaints in a follow-up study of a Dutch PCOS population. Hum Reprod 2001;16:556.

8 Wang ET, Cirillo PM, Vittinghoff E, Bibbins-Domingo K, Cohn BA, Cedars MI: Menstrual irregularity and cardiovascular mortality. J Clin Endocrinol Metab 2011;96:E114.

9 de Groot PCM, Dekkers OM, Romijn JA, Dieben SWM, Helmerhorst FM: PCOS, coronary heart disease, stroke and the influence of obesity: a systematic review and meta-analysis. Hum Reprod Update 2011;17:495.

10 Lambrinoudaki I: Cardiovascular risk in postmenopausal women with the polycystic ovary syndrome. Maturitas 2011;68:13.

11 Ouyang P, Vaidya D, Dobs A, Golden SH, Szklo M, Heckbert SR, Kopp P, Gapstur SM: Sex hormone levels and subclinical atherosclerosis in postmenopausal women: the multi-ethnic study of atherosclerosis. Atherosclerosis 2009;204:255.

12 Toulis KA, Goulis DG, Mintziori G, Kintiraki E, Eukarpidis E, Mouratoglou SA, Pavlaki A, Stergianos S, Poulasouchidou M, Tzellos TG, Makedos A, Chourdakis M, Tarlatzis BC: Meta-analysis of cardiovascular disease risk markers in women with polycystic ovary syndrome. Hum Reprod Update 2011;17:741.
13 Wild RA, Carmina E, Diamanti-Kandarakis E, Dokras A, Escobar-Morreale HF, Futterweit W, Lobo R, Norman RJ, Talbott E, Dumesic DA: Assessment of cardiovascular risk and prevention of cardiovascular disease in women with the polycystic ovary syndrome: a consensus statement by the Androgen Excess and Polycystic Ovary Syndrome (AE-PCOS) Society. J Clin Endocrinol Metab 2010;95:2038.
14 Kelly CJ, Speirs A, Gould GW, Petrie JR, Lyall H, Connell JM: Altered vascular function in young women with polycystic ovary syndrome. J Clin Endocrinol Metab 2002;87:742.
15 Diamanti-Kandarakis E, Spina G, Kouli C, Migdalis I: Increased endothelin-1 levels in women with polycystic ovary syndrome and the beneficial effect of metformin therapy. J Clin Endocrinol Metab 2001;86:4666.
16 Bentley-Lewis R, Seely E, Dunaif A: Ovarian hypertension: polycystic ovary syndrome. Endocrinol Metab Clin North Am 2011;40:433.
17 Armanini D, Castello R, Scaroni C, Bonanni G, Faccini G, Pellati D, Bertoldo A, Fiore C, Moghetti P: Treatment of polycystic ovary syndrome with spironolactone plus licorice. Eur J Obstet Gynecol Reprod Biol 2007;131:61.
18 Valkenburg O, Steegers-Theunissen RP, Smedts HP, Dallinga-Thie GM, Fauser BC, Westerveld EH, Laven JS: A more atherogenic serum lipoprotein profile is present in women with polycystic ovary syndrome: a case-control study. J Clin Endocrinol Metab 2008;93:470.
19 Fauser BC, Tarlatzis BC, Rebar RW, et al: Consensus on women's health aspects of polycystic ovary syndrome (PCOS): the Amsterdam ESHRE/ASRM-Sponsored 3rd PCOS Consensus Workshop Group. Fertil Steril 2012;97:28.
20 Rossi G, Boscaro M, Ronconi V, Funder JW: Aldosterone as a cardiovascular risk factor. Trends Endocrinol Metab 2005;16:104.
21 Cascella T, Palomba S, Tauchmanovà L, Manguso F, Di Biase S, Labella D, Giallauria F, Vigorito C, Colao A, Lombardi G, Orio F: Serum aldosterone concentration and cardiovascular risk in women with polycystic ovarian syndrome. J Clin Endocrinol Metab 2006;91:439522.
22 Bajuk-Studen K, Šebeštjen M, Pfeifer M, Preželj J: Influence of spironolactone treatment on endothelial function in non-obese women with polycystic ovary syndrome. Eur J Endocrinol 2011;164:389.
23 Davies JI, Band M, Morris A, Struthers AD: Spironolactone impairs endothelial function and heart rate variability in patients with type 2 diabetes. Diabetologia 2004;47:1687.
24 Nitsche K, Ehrmann DA: Obstructive sleep apnea and metabolic dysfunction in polycystic ovary syndrome. Best Pract Res Clin Endocrinol Metab 2010;24:717.
25 Tasali E, Chapotot F, Leproult L, Whitmore H, Ehrmann DA: Treatment of obstructive sleep apnea improves cardiometabolic function in young obese women with polycystic ovary syndrome. J Clin Endocrinol Metab 2011;96:365.
26 Deanfield JE, Halcox JP, Rabelink TJ: Endothelial function and dysfunction. Circulation 2007;115:1285.
27 Kim J, Montagnani M, Kon Koh K, Quon MJ: Reciprocal relationships between insulin resistance and endothelial dysfunction. Molecular and pathophysiological mechanisms. Circulation 2006;113:1888.
28 Paradisi G, Steinberg HO, Hempfling A, Cronin J, Hook G, Shepard MK, Baron AD: Polycystic ovary syndrome is associated with endothelial dysfunction. Circulation 2001;103:1410.
29 Kravariti M, Naka KK, Kalantaridou SN, Kazakos N, Katsouras CS, Makrigiannakis A, Paraskevaidis EA, Chrousos GP, Tsatsoulis A, Michalis LK: Predictors of endothelial dysfunction in young women with polycystic ovary syndrome. J Clin Endocrinol Metab 2005;90:5088.
30 Moran LJ, Noakes M, Clifton PM, Tomlinson L, Galletly C, Norman RJ: Dietary composition in restoring reproductive and metabolic physiology in overweight women with polycystic ovary syndrome. J Clin Endocrinol Metab 2003;88:812.
31 Mosca L: Guidelines for prevention of cardiovascular disease in women: a summary of recommendations. Prev Cardiol 2007;10(suppl 4):19.
32 Diamanti-Kandarakis E, Alexandraki K, Protogerou A, Piperi C, Papamichael C, Aessopos A, Lekakis J, Mavrikakis M: Metformin administration improves endothelial function in women with polycystic ovary syndrome. Eur J Endocrinol 2005;152:749.
33 Orio F Jr, Palomba S, Cascella T, De Simone B, Manguso F, Savastano S, Russo T, Tolino A, Zullo F, Lombardi G, Azziz R, Colao A: Improvement in endothelial structure and function after metformin treatment in young normal-weight women with polycystic ovary syndrome: results of a 6-month study. J Clin Endocrinol Metab 2005;90:6072.

34 Azziz R, Ehrmann D, Legro RS, Whitcomb RW, Hanley R, Fereshetian AG, O'Keefe M, Ghazzi MN, PCOS/Troglitazone Study Group: Troglitazone improves ovulation and hirsutism in the polycystic ovary syndrome: a multicenter, double blind, placebo-controlled trial. J Clin Endocrinol Metab 2001; 86:1626.
35 Tarkun I, Cetinarslan B, Türemen E, Sahin T, Cantürk Z, Komsuoglu B: Effect of rosiglitazone on insulin resistance, C-reactive protein and endothelial function in non-obese young women with polycystic ovary syndrome. Eur J Endocrinol 2005; 153:115.
36 Jensterle M, Šebeštjen M, Janež A, Prezelj J, Kocjan T, Keber I, Pfeifer M: Improvement of endothelial function with metformin and rosiglitazone treatment in women with polycystic ovary syndrome. Eur J Endocrinol 2008;159:399.
37 Mancini F, Cianciosi A, Persico N, Facchinetti F, Busacchi P, Battaglia C: Drospirenone and cardiovascular risk in lean and obese polycystic ovary syndrome patients: a pilot study. Am J Obstet Gynecol 2010;202:169.
38 Sathyapalan T, Atkin S: Review topic on mechanisms in endocrinology – recent advances in the cardiovascular aspects of polycystic ovary syndrome. Eur J Endocrinol 2012;166:575.
39 Pontikis C, Yavropoulou MP, Toulis KA, Kotsa K, Kazakos K, Papazisi A, Gotzamani-Psarakou A, Yovos JG: The incretin effect and secretion in obese and lean women with polycystic ovary syndrome: a pilot study. J Womens Health (Larchmt) 2011;20: 971.
40 Elkind-Hirsch K, Marrioneaux O, Bhushan M, Vernor D, Bhushan R: Comparison of single and combined treatment with exenatide and metformin on menstrual cyclicity in overweight women with polycystic ovary syndrome. J Clin Endocrinol Metab 2008;93:2670.

Marija Pfeifer, MD, PhD
Department of Endocrinology, Diabetes and Metabolic Diseases
University Medical Centre Ljubljana
Zaloska 7
SI–1525 Ljubljana (Slovenia)
Tel. +386 1 522 3122, E-Mail misa.pfeifer@kclj.si

Macut D, Pfeifer M, Yildiz BO, Diamanti-Kandarakis E (eds): Polycystic Ovary Syndrome. Novel Insights into Causes and Therapy. Front Horm Res. Basel, Karger, 2013, vol 40, pp 83–102

Insulin Sensitizers in Polycystic Ovary Syndrome

Renato Pasquali · Alessandra Gambineri

Division of Endocrinology, Department of Clinical Medicine, S. Orsola-Malpighi Hospital, University Alma Mater Studiorum, Bologna, Italy

Abstract

From the conceptual point of view, there are several reasons to expect that improvement of insulin sensitivity may produce several benefits in the treatment of a complex disorder like polycystic ovary syndrome (PCOS), including a decrease in insulin and androgen levels, improvement of metabolic comorbidities, and, finally, improved ovulation and fertility. This can be achieved with the help of specific agents, particularly metformin and thiazolidinediones. They may ease the suffering of women with PCOS because insulin resistance and hyperinsulinemia appear to be major contributors to the pathophysiology of the syndrome.

Insulin sensitizers are compounds positively influencing insulin sensitivity at target cells. This can be achieved in different ways, and all of the sensitizers are involved in the control of major pathways regulating insulin action at cellular levels, particularly in insulin-sensitive tissues such as liver, muscles and adipose tissue. Their efficacy can be measured in their ability to improve glucose metabolism; therefore, their primary role has been extensively investigated in the treatment of type 2 diabetes (T2D). The interest in polycystic ovary syndrome (PCOS) started several decades ago when it was firstly defined that most women with this disorder were characterized by the presence of some degree of insulin resistance and associated hyperinsulinemia [1]. Subsequently, a growing list of basic and clinical studies supported the notion that insulin may act as a true gonadotropic hormone, thereby participating in the regulation of ovarian steroidogenesis and granulosa cell function levels [2, 3]. A further step delineated that insulin sensitizers, particularly metformin, may add significant benefits to the treatment of PCOS by decreasing insulin resistance and improving glucose metabolism, by reducing serum androgen levels, improving anovulation and, possibly, infertility.

Insulin sensitizers are a group of therapeutic agents that may ease the suffering of women with PCOS, because insulin resistance and hyperinsulinemia appear to be major contributors to the pathophysiology of the syndrome. This chapter will deal with the rationale of using insulin sensitizers in women with PCOS, review major mechanisms of action, and summarize major studies on these drugs in the treatment of this disorder.

The Rationale for Using Insulin Sensitizers in PCOS

From the conceptual point of view, there are several reasons for expecting that improvement of insulin sensitivity may produce several benefits in the treatment of a complex disorder like PCOS. First, compensatory hyperinsulinemia can be reduced, which in turn is expected to reduce circulating androgens, and increase sex hormone-binding globulin (SHBG) synthesis, thereby reducing free androgen fraction availability in peripheral tissues. Second, it may ameliorate glucose intolerance states, and the onset of T2D could be theoretically delayed in susceptible individuals, if not completely prevented. Third, improved insulin sensitivity and reduced insulin concentrations can increase fertility rates in otherwise infertile or hypofertile women. Fourth, by decreasing insulin-mediated androgen excess and tissue availability of free androgens, through both peripheral and central [2, 3] mechanisms, most of the related signs and symptoms could be at least partially improved. Fifth, in this way the metabolic syndrome and other associated risk factors for cardiovascular disease may be attenuated. Most of these actions have been widely discussed in recent extensive reviews [4–6].

Insulin-Sensitizing Agents

Insulin sensitizers are a group of therapeutic agents that may ease the suffering of women with PCOS, because insulin resistance and hyperinsulinemia appear to be major contributors to the pathophysiology of the syndrome. This is a relatively new therapeutic approach targeting improvement of insulin resistance and aiming to modify the effect of hyperinsulinemia not only on classic insulin-sensitive tissues but on ovarian tissue as well. There are two families of insulin-sensitizing agents that have been used in clinical trials for the management of PCOS. One is the family of biguanides, in particular metformin, and the other the family of thiazolidinediones (TZDs) for which there are fewer studies, partly related to their restrictional use by international agencies.

Historically, metformin was first used in women with PCOS in 1994 to investigate the role of insulin resistance in the pathogenesis of the syndrome. In the original paper by Velasquez and colleagues [7], menses became more frequent with metformin use and there was a significant improvement in androgen blood levels. However, the authors found a small but significant decrease in bodyweight, so that it was impossible to conclude that metabolic benefits were accounted for solely by improvements in insulin sensitivity. In 1996, studies in which women with PCOS received troglitazone (the first available TZD for human treatment) demonstrated that it decreased androgen levels in parallel with the increase in insulin sensitivity, without changes in bodyweight [7]. Since then, numerous studies have been published, particularly on metformin, and several meta-analyses provide adequate information on the role of insulin sensitizers in the management of PCOS. Nevertheless, how metformin and TZDs should be used in the treatment of PCOS still remains a matter of intense debate.

Metformin: Mechanisms of Action

Metformin has pleiotropic actions on several tissues sensitive to the primary effect of insulin or affected by insulin resistance, such as the liver, the skeletal muscles, the adipose tissue, the endothelium and the ovaries [8]. They will be summarized below.

The primary function of metformin, which has been confirmed in both animal models and clinical studies, is to decrease hepatic glucose production mainly by inhibiting gluconeogenesis. Several mechanisms have been proposed to explain this effect, including changes in enzyme activity or a reduction in hepatic uptake of gluconeogenic substrates. The mechanisms potentially involve the direct inhibition of gluconeogenic enzymes (e.g. phospho-enolpyruvate carboxykinase, fructose-1,6-bisphosphatase, and glucose-6-phosphatase), the reduced hepatic uptake of substrates for gluconeogenesis, the increased phosphorylation of insulin receptor substrates (IRS)-1 and -2, and the inhibition of mitochondrial respiration. Simultaneously, metformin stimulates glucose entry into the liver and glycolysis through activation of glycolytic enzymes, such as hexokinase and pyruvate kinase. The molecular target of metformin has been investigated for many years, but for the first time Zhou at al. [9] reported that the activation of the AMP protein kinase (AMPK) was closely associated with the pleiotropic actions of metformin. Interestingly, AMPK is a phylogenetically conserved serine/threonine protein kinase, viewed as a fuel gauge monitoring systemic and cellular energy status, and which plays a crucial role in protecting cellular functions under energy-restricted conditions. There is evidence that AMPK activation by metformin may be secondary to its effect on the mitochondria, performed through specific inhibition of the respiratory chain complex 1, although the exact mechanism still remains unknown. The demonstration that respiratory chain complex 1 but not AMPK is the primary target for metformin was strengthened by showing that the metabolic effect of the drug is preserved in liver-specific AMPK-deficient mice.

In addition to the suppression of endogenous glucose production, metformin has been shown to improve lipid metabolism. Notably, metformin suppresses acetyl-CoA carboxylase activity, an important rate-controlling enzyme for the synthesis of malonyl-CoA, a critical precursor in the biosynthesis of fatty acids and a potent inhibitor of mitochondrial fatty acid oxidation, therefore leading to decreased fatty acid synthesis, and increased mitochondrial fatty acid oxidation. As a consequence, metformin regulates the partitioning of fatty acids between oxidative and biosynthetic pathways. The positive impact of metformin on lipid metabolism is supported by the fact that the drug has beneficial effects on fatty liver by reversing hepatic steatosis not only in experimental animals, but also in humans. The effects of metformin on hepatic lipid content are consistent with an increase in fatty acid oxidation and inhibition of lipogenesis, presumably mediated by AMPK activation. In addition, AMPK suppresses the expression of several lipogenic genes (such as fatty acid synthase-FAS, etc.), participates in the regulation of lipogenesis by downregulating other genes and by inhibiting proteolitic processing and transcriptional activity upon AMPK-mediated phosphorylation at Ser372. Stimulation of AMPK has emerged as a putative key mediator of the hepatic actions of metformin on gluconeogenesis and lipogenesis.

Metformin increases insulin-mediated glucose uptake not only in the liver, but also in the visceral fat, thereby increasing the re-esterification of free fatty acids (FFAs), reducing lipolysis and FFA delivery to the liver [5, 7].

Although the adipose tissue is not considered a major site of metformin's action, there are studies showing that metformin may, independent of insulin action, increase preadipocyte glucose transport and utilization, mitochondrial and peroxisomal fatty acid β-oxidation and basal lipolysis, particularly in the visceral adipose tissue [5]. Some studies have shown that metformin seems to inhibit the TNF-α induced lipolysis in primary rat adipocytes, which suggests that it may contribute to insulin sensitization through the decrease of systemic FFA levels. In addition, other studies have shown that metformin may counteract adipose tissue expansion through direct inhibition of adipogenesis in pre-adipocytes, although these effects have not been demonstrated in vivo. Interestingly, there are data supporting the concept that metformin may selectively favor a reduction of visceral fat in the long-term, although this has been a matter of debate.

In the skeletal muscles, which account for more than 80% of insulin-stimulated glucose uptake, metformin has been reported to promote a moderate increase in glucose uptake [5]. In cultures of insulin-resistant skeletal muscle cells, metformin has also been found to restore the reduction in IRS-1 phosphorylation and phosphatidyl inositol 3 kinase activity. In humans, chronic treatment with metformin reduces lipid accumulation in human skeletal muscle tissue. By means of these effects on lipid metabolism, it is suggested that metformin may contribute to improved insulin sensitivity and insulin-stimulated glucose uptake, although the potential efficacy of metformin to improve insulin resistance in the muscles needs to be further investigated.

Metformin may also exert its beneficial metabolic action in part through the modulation of the incretin axis [8]. Original studies in rats showed that metformin reduced dipeptidyl peptidase-4 activity, and acutely increased glucagon-like peptide-1 (GLP-1) plasma levels in both rats and humans, and chronically in humans. More recently, these effects have been confirmed; however, it was shown that metformin may also modulate multiple components of the incretin axis, including not only the stimulatory effect of GLP-1, but also by enhancing the expression of GLP-1 receptor and related insulinotropic receptors, through a mechanism that is dependent on peroxisome proliferator-activated receptor-α (PPARα).

Apart from its action on classic insulin sensitive tissues, metformin also has a direct effect at the ovarian level [3, 7, 8]. Its beneficial effects are partly based on the alleviation of excess insulin. Insulin was shown to directly stimulate several steroidogenic enzymes in the ovary, such as CYP(cytochrome P450)17, 3β-hydroxysteroid dehydrogenase (3β-HSD) and the steroidogenic acute regulatory protein (StAR) protein, and, in this way, the gonadotropic action of insulin synergizes that of lutein hormone (LH). By improving insulin sensitivity, metformin reduces CYP17 activity. Furthermore, metformin suppresses androstenedione production by a direct effect on ovarian theca cells and decreases FSH (follicle-stimulating hormone)-stimulated 3β-HSD, StAR, CYP11A1 and aromatase activities in both rat granulosa cells and women with PCOS [5]. Although the molecular pathways whereby metformin acts directly on the ovary remain partly elusive, it has been demonstrated that metformin treatment increased AMPK activity in rat granulosa cells, leading to subsequent reduction of steroid synthesis. However, it is still unclear whether this effect is AMPK dependent or not. Interestingly, metformin has been shown to reduce the risks of abortion in women with PCOS at high risk of pregnancy and neonatal complications by increasing some factors needed for implantation and pregnancy safekeeping, such as insulin-growth factor-binding protein-1 and glycodelin levels, or uterine artery blood flow. By contrast, metformin reduces factors increasing the risk of abortion, such as endometrial androgen receptor expression, PAI-1 (plasminogen-activator inhibitor-1) levels and plasma ET-1 (endothelin-1). Most of these effects are probably mediated by the metformin-induced improvement in insulin sensitivity [4, 5].

Metformin: Clinical Effects

Clinical benefits of metformin in women with PCOS include: (a) improved menses cyclicity, (b) anovulation, (c) pregnancy outcomes, (d) endometrial function, (e) hyperandrogenemia, (f) obesity and fat distribution, (g) metabolic alterations, (h) cardiovascular risk factors, (i) insulin resistance and hyperinsulinemia, and (j) chronic inflammation. These effects have recently been summarized in several reviews to which the reader can refer for detailed information [4–7].

Menses, Ovulation, Infertility and Pregnancy Outcomes

Here, we will summarize and update the main findings supporting the clinical and biological efficacy of metformin in women with PCOS. The majority of studies have shown that, in most PCOS women, metformin may significantly improve menstrual cycles and ovulation rates, both spontaneous and clomiphene citrate (CC) induced or FSH induced, although discordant data have been reported in some studies. This is particularly evident in studies using metformin for several weeks before CC was administered. In this case, metformin seems to act as a sensitizer for CC action. In their meta-analysis performed in 2003, including all controlled trials available at that time, Lord et al. [10] reported that metformin was effective in achieving ovulation in women with PCOS with an odds ratios of 3.88 (95% confidence interval, 2.25–6.69) when metformin was compared to placebo and 4.41 (95% confidence interval, 2.37–8.22) when metformin plus clomiphene was compared to clomiphene alone. Soon after, a systematic review by Kashyap et al. [11] reported the same conclusions and suggested that metformin would be effective for the achievement of pregnancy when compared to CC. This appeared to be particularly evident in CC-resistant PCOS women.

In the following years, many meta-analyses or randomized controlled trials (RCTs) have been published, and the relevant findings are summarized below. The highest level of evidence on the use of metformin versus placebo or no treatment is evident in the Cochrane systematic review by Tang et al. [12] who performed a meta-analysis of RCTs comparing metformin with placebo or no treatment in women with PCOS, which showed that metformin improves ovulation rate and clinical pregnancy rate but not live birth rate per woman. The same Cochrane systematic review [12] also compared metformin versus CC in women with PCOS and found a reduced ovulation rate per cycle and reduced clinical pregnancy rate, but no difference in the live birth rate with metformin in women with PCOS in general. In a subanalysis of women grouped according to BMI values, it was found that women with PCOS with a BMI >30 had a lower ovulation rate, clinical pregnancy and live birth rates while taking metformin, whereas no effect was present in those with lower BMI values. Two RCTs comparing metformin versus CC in women with PCOS, published after Tang's Cochrane review [13, 14], confirmed that CC was superior to metformin overall for ovulation induction in women with PCOS, and for women with PCOS with a BMI >30, whilst the RCT data are conflicting in women with PCOS with a BMI <30. In addition, a recent meta-analysis of RCTs comparing metformin versus CC in non-obese PCOS women demonstrated no difference in clinical pregnancy rate or live birth rate, although the results should be interpreted with caution because the results are based on statistical heterogeneous data. The most recent systematic reviews and meta-analyses of RCTs that have compared the combination of metformin plus CC versus CC alone in various classes of women with PCOS included women with PCOS with variable BMI lower or higher than 30, and those who were CC naïve or resistant [15]. Metformin combined with CC had higher ovulation, pregnancy and live birth rates without statistical heterogeneity compared to CC alone only in CC-resistant PCOS. Therefore, the addition of metformin to CC appears to be more beneficial in CC-resistant women with PCOS than persisting with more cycles of CC alone. The most current systematic reviews and meta-analyses of RCTs comparing the combination of metformin plus CC versus metformin alone in PCOS demonstrated a higher ovulation rate per patient, pregnancy rate, and live birth rate with metformin combined with CC. A number of systematic reviews and meta-analyses of RCTs have found no evidence of any benefit when metformin is added to laparoscopic ovarian drilling, gonadotropin ovulation induction with timed intercourse, or IVF/ICSI treatment (e.g. ovarian hyperstimulation syndrome) [5, 15].

Hyperandrogenism

In women with PCOS, the majority of studies have demonstrated that metformin decreases fasting and glucose-stimulated insulin, testosterone and LH levels [4, 5]. Some other studies have also reported that the degree of hirsutism was attenuated, although this does not represent a common and significant finding. Although mechanistic studies on all potential mechanisms responsible for metformin effects on the gonadal axis do not permit conclusive information, it is nonetheless generally accepted that the effects of metformin on hyperandrogenism may depend on the decrease in circulating insulin and improved insulin sensitivity, increased SHBG levels, which in turn decrease bioavailable free testosterone, and, possibly, decreased IGF-1, due to increased IGF-1-binding protein-1 [4].

Excess Weight and Obesity, the Metabolic Syndrome, Insulin Resistance, and Cardiovascular Risk Factors

As a monotherapy, metformin does not reduce bodyweight, although some studies have reported some marginal benefit [16]. By contrast, it has been shown that in combination with lifestyle intervention, metformin can favor some additional benefit on weight loss and reduce abdominal fat in abdominally obese women with PCOS. These effects can be associated with more benefit on insulin levels and insulin resistance [7]. On the other hand, large RCTs should be performed to confirm and expand these findings, and possibly to investigate individual metabolic, hormonal and ovulatory responsiveness.

Metformin obviously has important effects on the parameters of the metabolic syndrome. In particular, in their meta-analysis, Lord et al. [10] reported a significant decrease in circulating fasting insulin levels. In small controlled studies using the clamp technique, a significant but incomplete correction of insulin resistance was also found, particularly in obese individuals [7]. The effects of metformin on lipids were investigated in some studies and, although a significant improvement was observed in both triglyceride and HDL cholesterol concentrations, a great variability was nonetheless described among groups and individuals. Other studies showed an improvement of proinflammatory markers, such as PAI-1, endothelin, and C reactive protein [4].

As mentioned above, metformin should always be used in addition to hypocaloric diet or lifestyle intervention in overweight or obese PCOS women. The theoretical basis for this clinical approach in PCOS should be substantially the same as for T2D, as recommended by the latest guidelines for treatment of T2D. Moreover, as for T2D [17], it is theoretically possible that lifestyle intervention and metformin could even help to prevent the development of PCOS, although this cannot be defined without appropriate longitudinal studies. Unfortunately, very few studies combining metformin with lifestyle intervention have been performed, particularly in obese PCOS women. In one placebo- and case-controlled study [cited in reference 7] performed to evaluate the additive efficacy of metformin upon a low calorie diet regimen in abdominally obese women with PCOS, we found a greater reduction of bodyweight and abdominal fat, particularly the visceral depots, and a more consistent decrease in serum insulin, testosterone and leptin concentrations after metformin (850 mg/orally, twice daily) administration when compared to placebo. Moreover, these changes were associated with a significant improvement of hirsutism and menses abnormalities. Overall, these data indicate that metformin may produce significant additional benefits to weight loss regimens.

Metformin: Side Effects

The most common adverse effects of metformin are gastrointestinal (diarrhea, nausea, flatulence, dyspepsia, etc.). These effects occur in 10–50% of patients receiving metformin therapy but are usually transient and resolve within a few days to weeks after the initiation of therapy, and their severity can be lessened by employing a gradual titration schedule [4]. Metformin therapy may rarely cause malabsorption of vitamin B12 in the distal ileum in some patients. An increased risk of vitamin B12 deficiency has been associated with increasing patient age, current dose and duration of metformin use. Very rare metformin-associated megaloblastic anemias have been reported. Lactic acidosis is a very rare side effect of metformin; however, clinical conditions such as renal dysfunction or organ hypoxia or alcohol abuse should represent a contraindication for metformin.

Metformin Pharmacokinetics

Metformin is a biguanide developed from galegine, a guanidine derivative found in Galega officinalis. Chemically, it is a hydrophilic base which exists at physiological pH as the cationic species (>99.9%). Consequently, its passive diffusion through cell membranes should be very limited. The fractional oral bioavailability of metformin is

55 ± 16%, and it is absorbed predominately by the small intestine. After oral administration of metformin at doses of 500–1,500 mg to healthy volunteers, absorption was not complete (20–30% of the oral dose was recovered from feces) possibly due to an active, saturable absorption process, and the absolute oral bioavailability was 33–55% [18]. After intravenous administration of metformin at doses of 250–1,000 mg to healthy volunteers, the terminal half-life of the drug was 1.5–4.5 h, and 79–100% of the dose was excreted in urine via active renal tubular secretion. Metformin does not bind to human plasma proteins [18]. Metabolism of metformin was suggested in humans, based on its incomplete recovery in the urine after its intravenous administration and on a further study in which 20% of the dose was not accounted for. Studies in vitro incubating metformin with the 9,000 g supernatant fractions of livers from male Sprague-Dawley rats showed that approximately 20% of the added metformin (10 μg) disappeared after 30-min incubation [cited in reference 18]. This suggested that rat liver could metabolize metformin. However, the types of hepatic microsomal cytochrome P450 (CYP) isozymes responsible for the metabolism of metformin in humans and rats have not yet been identified. In a study performed to find out what types of CYP isozymes are responsible for the metabolism of metformin in rats, it was found that CYP2C11, 2D1 and 3A1/2 were involved in the metabolism of metformin in male Sprague-Dawley rats [cited in reference 18]. Obviously, it would clearly be of importance to determine the CYP isozymes involved in metformin pharmacokinetics in humans.

Metformin is excreted unchanged in urine. The elimination half-life of metformin during multiple dosages in patients with good renal function is approximately 5 h. The population mean renal clearance and apparent total clearance after oral administration of metformin have been estimated to be 510 ± 130 and 1,140 ± 330 ml/min, respectively, in healthy subjects and diabetic patients with good renal function. The oral absorption, hepatic uptake and renal excretion of metformin are mediated largely by organic cation transporter-1 (OCT1), as reported in a previous paragraph.

The clinical effects of metformin develop slowly over at least several days of treatment, and the range of plasma concentrations over a dosage interval depends upon the formulation without any significant effect on the clinical response. The plasma concentrations of metformin have been recorded in a number of studies with most emphasis on the concentrations which are not associated with lactic acidosis (average concentrations at steady state over a dosage interval values up to 250 mg/ml), and, overall, these estimated values are consistent with a tentative recommendation for clinical use. The control and monitoring of the dosage of metformin are contentious areas; however, it is generally recommended that metformin should be administered initially at a low rate in order to mitigate the adverse gastrointestinal effects. In addition, doses should be increased to a maximum of 2,550–3,000 mg daily in patients with good renal function although lower dosage may be sufficient, and the dose of metformin should be individualized because of inter-subject variation in bioavailability and response. Notably, the plasma concentrations of metformin are not monitored in current clinical practice, although monitoring the plasma concentrations could also be valuable in patients who fail to respond. Support for monitoring the plasma concentrations comes from the observation that the clinical response to metformin increases with increasing doses and, further, that a higher dose of metformin is required in patients with higher pretreatment fasting blood glucose levels. Intuitively, all these aspects should be considered in women with PCOS.

Metformin: Are the Effects Dose Dependent?

Worldwide, extremely varying target doses of metformin have been used in studies on women with PCOS, mostly ranging from 1,500 to 2,550 mg/day. However, to date, no dose-finding study is available for a PCOS population, therapeutic regimens are not well standardized in clinical practice, and heterogeneous protocols have been reported in published studies. A dose-response effect of immediate release metformin in obese PCOS women has been suggested, based on the lack of changes in insulin levels and indirect indices of insulin resistance on doses of 500 mg t.i.d., although improved efficacy was observed when 850 mg t.i.d. were administered. On the other hand, based on studies performed in patients with T2D, it has been suggested that maximal benefits may be obtained at the upper limits of the recommended dosage. Again, there is no standardization on how long metformin should be administered in women with PCOS, unlike what happens in the treatment or prevention of T2D. In addition, it is still unknown whether metformin should be used as a symptomatic therapy for infertility and hyperandrogenism, or rather as a chronic treatment to prevent late-onset comorbidities. Interestingly, recent data obtained in a non-insulin-resistant PCOS population showed that, after long-term metformin treatment, drug suspension was followed by a rapid reversion of its beneficial effect on peripheral insulin sensitivity measured by the hyperinsulinemic euglycemic clamp technique, which was followed by a worsening of hyperandrogenism and menstrual cyclicity [4]. In addition, it has been shown that the withdrawal of metformin treatment was followed within 3 months by a significant reversal toward a pretreatment hyperandrogenic hyperinsulinemic state in non-obese adolescents with hirsutism, oligomenorrhea, and a history of precocious pubarche [cited in reference 18].

A recent study performed in a multicenter Italian cohort, including approximately 250 women with PCOS treated with different doses of metformin (1,000/1,500/1,700 mg daily) administered for 6 months, examined whether doses of metformin could influence major outcomes, such as menstrual cycles and insulin changes [manuscript under revision]. The data confirmed an overall positive effect of metformin on clinical and endocrine-metabolic features of PCOS. The efficacy of metformin seemed to be independent of the dosage in the different clusters of basal BMI, but when patients were stratified on the basis of their fasting insulin levels, scattered differences in the effects of the different dosages were found in some of the outcome measures. Interestingly, patients who were responders to metformin treatment (based on the increase of at least 2 cycles/year) did not differ significantly from non-responder patients regarding outcome measures. These findings seem to support the concept that metformin efficacy in women with PCOS is likely to be independent of the dose.

Metformin: Factors Involved in Predicting Response

Knowledge regarding the predictors for metformin response is crucial because their identification could guide clinicians to the best individualized treatment to improve metformin's efficacy. In general, the beneficial effects of metformin may vary according to the clinical characteristics of each patient. First, the gastrointestinal absorption of the drug ranges from 20 to 30% and is dose-dependent, proportionally greater for a dose of 500 mg than for 1,500 mg, as transport occurs exclusively via the paracellular route and is saturable [4]. This mechanism could be responsible for a tangible reduction in the difference of the circulating concentrations of the drug between users of lower and higher metformin dosages. Notably, in experimental animals it has been shown that the degree of insulin resistance itself may induce significant variations in the hepatic or renal clearance of metformin [4].

Studies performed in women with PCOS have shown that metformin may produce some benefit irrespective of their bodyweight or degree of insulin resistance [4]. By contrast, other studies supported the concept that the drug may be more effective in insulin-resistant PCOS patients with low BMI, although this needs to be confirmed by further studies. Whether the pattern of fat distribution may predict responsiveness is also contradictory. A recent analysis of previous randomized controlled studies [19] provided evidence for a significantly different change of ongoing pregnancy between PCOS women receiving metformin if they were young (<28 years) and had high waist-to-hip ratio values. Baseline normal or borderline androstenedione (but not testosterone) blood levels, together with fasting insulin values, were shown to predict menses restoration in one study, suggesting that the lower the hyperandrogenic state the higher the probability of improving menses.

Specific genetic variation may also be associated with response to metformin. A recent study has shown that a serine-threonine kinase gene expressed in the liver, STK11 (formerly known as LKB1), is required in the liver to control blood glucose levels. STK11 phosphorylates and activates AMPK, and is also a tumor suppressor gene implicated in the etiology of Peutz-Jeghers syndrome [4]. The deletion of STK11 in the liver of adult mice resulted in hyperglycemia with increased gluconeogenic and lipogenic gene expression, and its presence was required for metformin efficacy. Recently, data from the Pregnancy in PCOS trial indicated that a polymorphism of STK11 was associated with a significantly decreased chance of ovulation in PCOS patients treated with metformin, which suggests that this gene may be involved in metformin action [20].

The preferential action of metformin on hepatocytes is due to the predominant expression of OCT1, which has been shown to be higher than in other tissues, reaching higher micromolar concentrations in the peripheral periportal area. Furthermore, deletion of the Oct1 [SLC22A1 (solute carrier family 22 member 1)] gene in mice dramatically reduces metformin uptake in hepatocytes, and human subjects carrying polymorphisms of the SLC22A1 gene display an impaired effect of metformin on lowering blood glucose levels [21]. There is also evidence that polymorphisms in the OCT1, which is expressed in the liver, are associated with changes in pharmacokinetic/pharmacodynamic responses to metformin. Although OCT1 plays a role in the hepatic uptake of metformin, its role in the therapeutic effects of the drug, which involve activation of AMPK, is still unknown. Since human OCT1 is highly polymorphic, information on whether OCT1 plays a role in the action of metformin and whether individuals with OCT1 polymorphisms have a reduced response to the drug may be of interest. Seven non-synonymous polymorphisms of OCT1 that exhibited reduced uptake of metformin were also identified. Notably, OCT1-420del had reduced activity for metformin. In addition, clinical studies performed by the same authors referred to above [21] showed that the effects of metformin in glucose tolerance tests were significantly lower in individuals carrying reduced function polymorphisms of OCT1, thus suggesting that OCT1 is important for metformin's therapeutic action, and that genetic variations in OCT1 may contribute to variations in response to the drug. In a recent study performed in a large sample of diabetic subjects, to evaluate the effect of genetic variations of OCT1 on the trough steady-state plasma concentration of metformin and hemoglobin A1c (Hb1Ac), it was found that the mean trough steady-state metformin plasma concentration and the absolute decrease in Hb1Ac were highly and significantly correlated with the number of reduced function alleles in OCT1. These findings further support that OCT1 activity affects metformin steady-state pharmacokinetics, other than having a bearing on HbA1c during metformin treatment [23]. In addition, in a large cohort of women with PCOS treated with three different doses of metformin (500 mg b.i.d., 500 mg t.i.d., or 850 mg b.i.d.) for 6 months, we recently investigated the effectiveness of the treatment based on the OCT1 genotype. The prevalence of each variant in heterozygosis (four SNPs, R61C, G401S, G465R, and 420del) was 9.7, 2.8, 1.4, and 28.3%, respectively. One woman (0.7%) was homozygous for R61C and 4 (2.8%) for 420 del. With respect to the non-variant women, those presenting with polymorphisms (the variant group) did not show any significant differences in baseline clinical, hormonal and metabolic parameters. By contrast, the variant group had, with respect to the reference group, a significantly lower decrease in total cholesterol, triglycerides and insulin response to the oral glucose tolerance test after 6 months of metformin treatment. These data provide proof of the concept, in a clinical setting, that a genetic variation of OCT1 may be associated with heterogeneity in the metabolic response to metformin in PCOS women. Hopefully, the need for a pharmacogenomic approach to the use of metformin will emerge in the near future.

Thiazolidinediones

TZDs are selective ligands of the nuclear transcription factor PPARγ, which is expressed most abundantly in adipose tissue, pancreatic β-cells, vascular endothelium, and macrophages [24]. The first TZD, troglitazone, was approved as a glucose-lowering therapy for patients with T2D in 1997. Troglitazone was subsequently withdrawn from the market in 2000, because of hepatotoxicity. Currently, the two available TZDs are rosiglitazone and pioglitazone. Recent concerns about the cardiovascular safety of rosiglitazone have led to some restriction in the use of the drug by international agencies. A recent review on this topic investigating the safety of pioglitazone and rosiglitazone under the headings of liver safety, cardiovascular safety, fluid retention, weight gain and bone fractures was based on a PubMed search of the years 1997 through June 2010 [25]. According to the conclusion of the expert, liver safety is no longer an issue with the TZDs. There are no significant differences between rosiglitazone and pioglitazone in fluid retention, weight gain and bone fractures. However, pioglitazone tends to be cardioprotective while rosiglitazone is cardiotoxic. There is no current justification for prescribing rosiglitazone.

Thiazolidinediones: Mechanisms of Action

TZDs represent a further class of drugs that decrease peripheral insulin resistance by enhancing insulin action in the skeletal muscle, liver and adipose tissues [26]. These agents are believed to work through binding and modulating the activity of a family of nuclear transcription factors termed PPAR. Improvement of insulin sensitivity by TZDs simultaneously decreases circulating blood insulin levels, thereby reducing the major factors responsible for androgen excess in women with PCOS, i.e. decreased SHBG concentrations (in this way they decrease free androgen availability) and increased ovarian theca cell steroidogenesis. Specifically, the PPARγ isoform could be considered as a fuel sensor linking energy metabolism and reproduction to inform cells on the energy status. Indeed, PPARγ can regulate the transcription and/or activity of different key regulators of energy homeostasis such as glucose or lipid regulators (PPARγ upregulated expression of glucose transporters, insulin receptor, IRS, fatty acid-binding protein, etc.). Activation of PPARγ by TZDs increases insulin sensitivity mainly in adipocytes and muscle cells, and also stimulates the differentiation of adipose cells. This may occur because of the ability of pioglitazone to enhance insulin sensitivity directly, by improving signaling through AKT and AS160. In addition, pioglitazone has been found to modify the transcriptional profile favoring insulin sensitivity in muscles of PCOS women by a coordinated upregulation of genes involved in mitochondrial oxidative phosphorylation and ribosomal protein biosynthesis. In another study, protein content, activity, and phosphorylation of glycogen synthase (GS) and its major upstream inhibitor, GS kinase (GSK)-3, were investigated in skeletal muscle biopsies from PCOS patients before and after treatment with pioglitazone. In fact, it was found that lower than normal insulin-mediated glucose disposal, measured by a clamp technique, in PCOS, was associated with a lower insulin-stimulated GS, and that this was partly explained by absent insulin-mediated dephosphorylation of GS at the NH2-terminal sites 2 + 2°, therefore suggesting that improvement of impaired insulin sensitivity may involve an improved insulin action on GS activity and dephosphorylation at NH2 terminal sites. Unlike what was previously suggested, it has been recently shown that the genetic mechanisms governing insulin resistance in skeletal muscle of PCOS patients in vivo may not be primary, but rather adaptive, since myotubes established from PCOS or control patients with or without pioglitazone treatment showed no significant differences between them, either at baseline or during acute insulin stimulation, although in vivo pioglitazone treatment significantly improved insulin sensitivity. Finally, the insulin-resistant state of PCOS has been found to be associated with a decreased glucose transporter GLUT4 expression in the insulin target tissues. A 6-month therapy with rosiglitazone resulted in marked improvement in adipose tissue GLUT4 mRNA expression in PCOS patients, which was more effective when compared with metformin.

In addition, the three PPAR isoforms (PPARα, PPARβ/δ, PPARγ) are expressed along the gonadotrope axis (central nervous system, pituitary gland and ovary) [26]. In the ovaries, the expression of PPARγ seems to be restricted to follicles, primarily to granulosa cells, although they can also be slightly expressed in theca cells and in the corpus luteum. After the LH surge, the PPARγ expression decreases in follicles. However, additional studies have shown that a PPARγ-independent action of TZDs cannot be excluded. Studies in ruminants have shown a direct effect of glucose or fatty acids on folliculogenesis; therefore, the ovulation rate was increased without modification of gonadotropin secretion as observed in the case of flushing. However, deletion of PPARγ did not modify folliculogenesis or ovulation rate in rodents, neither did it modify the number of corpus luteum, although a decrease in the number of embryos implanted was observed, probably due to a drop in progesterone secretion by the corpus luteum. In humans, linkage studies have rejected a genetic association between the PPARγ locus (3p25) and the birth of dizygotic twins.

Changes in PPARγ activation may also modify steroid secretion by granulosa and thecal cells. In vitro, it has been found that steroid secretions (androgens, progesterone, estradiol) were partially inhibited or stimulated by TZDs according to species or the status of the cell differentiation (follicular phase, before or after the preovulatory surge). In addition, TZDs have been found to stimulate progesterone secretion by a mixture of granulosa, theca, and stroma human cells obtained from premenopausal/perimenopausal patients at the time of oophorectomy, and to partially inhibit testosterone, progesterone and estradiol secretion by human granulosa cells (after hCG stimulation for in vitro fertilization), or by luteal-granulosa cells obtained from PCOS patients. Furthermore, in vitro studies have shown that TZDs may inhibit LH/insulin-stimulated androgen secretion by porcine thecal cells. The inhibiting effect of TZDs in human theca cells seems to be due more to a reduction in the activity of steroidogenic enzymes 3β-HSD and aromatase, rather than to an activation of PPARγ on the promoters of the genes encoding these enzymes. Improved ovarian insulin sensitivity by TZDs seems also to favor the restoration of steroidogenesis to a normal status. Indeed, the responsiveness to FSH in human granulosa cells obtained in PCOS patients was enhanced by insulin after improvement of insulin sensitivity by the pioglitazone treatment, which is consistent with the possibility that PCOS granulosa cells are insulin resistant and that this can be directly improved by pioglitazone. In addition, preliminary studies have shown that pioglitazone and rosiglitazone increased the level of insulin receptor and IRS-1 in human ovarian cells 2- to 3-fold. Interestingly, a further study found that the overactivation of the mitogen-activated protein/extracellular signal-regulated kinase MEK/ERK signaling pathway, which may play a role in regulating androgen biosynthesis in PCOS, can be reversed by pioglitazone, which again suggests that its action in the ovarian tissues may be partly independent of PPARγ activation.

Thiazolidinediones: Clinical Effects

TZDs consistently lower fasting and postprandial glucose concentration [25]. However, what drives the use of TZDs in PCOS is their action as insulin sensitizers. TZDs exert their insulin-sensitizing actions either directly (the 'fatty acid steal' hypothesis) or indirectly, by means of altered adipokine release, particularly adiponectin, thereby modulating insulin sensitivity outside adipose tissue. According to the 'fatty acid steal' hypothesis, TZDs promote fatty acid uptake and storage in adipose tissue. In this way, they increase adipo-tissue mass and spare other insulin-sensitive tissues such as skeletal muscle and the liver, and possibly pancreatic β-cells, from the harmful metabolic effects of high levels of FFAs. TZDs thus keep fat where it belongs.

The three placebo-controlled studies published so far on the effect of TZDs in PCOS [27–29] demonstrate that pioglitazone or rosiglitazone decrease fasting glucose and insulin levels, and the glucose and insulin response to glucose load, as AUC (i.e. the curve of concentration versus time). In addition, they reduce androgen levels, particularly free testosterone, ameliorate hirsutism, and improve ovulation rates. Overall, these data suggest that metformin and TZDs have similar hormonal and metabolic effects in PCOS. This suggestion has been confirmed by the several small RCTs that compared TZDs and metformin in PCOS [cited in reference 7]. When we add the high cost of TZDs to this awareness, we are justified in affirming that TZDs cannot be considered an indiscriminate alternative to metformin for the treatment of women with PCOS.

But what, then, is the indication for the use of TZDs in PCOS? One indication for the use of TZDs in PCOS, in substitution of or in addition to metformin, could be the condition of non-responsiveness to metformin. The utility of the addition of TZDs in women with PCOS who failed to respond to metformin is well documented in one study where the addition of pioglitazone to metformin in non-responder women to metformin itself was followed by a significant benefit on the metabolic parameters. In addition, in women on pioglitazone plus metformin, the occurrence of expected menses was 2-fold higher than in those on metformin alone. However, it should be taken into account that there are potential drawbacks to the addition of TZDs to metformin: the cessation of weight loss, particularly in dieting obese PCOS women, and the toxicity in pregnancy. TZDs, in fact, promote weight gain, mainly related to their mechanism of action as PPARγ ligands, but also to fluid retention [30]. In addition, rosiglitazone and pioglitazone have both been classified for pregnancy as category C, drugs with a toxic effect in studies in animal models, but with inadequate studies in humans. In animal models, in fact, treatment during mid-late gestation was associated with fetal death. Therefore, the addition of TZD to metformin should be contraindicated when weight loss is the main outcome of treatment, or when the desire for pregnancy is prevalent.

One of the causes of non-responsiveness to metformin is PCOS secondary to genetically determined severe insulin resistance. This condition, although rare, does exist and must be taken into account and adequately excluded in the initial evaluation of all patients with PCOS.

Metformin and Thiazolidinediones in PCOS: Comparative Studies

A recent meta-analysis to assess the effectiveness and safety of metformin versus TZDs (including pioglitazone and rosiglitazone) in the treatment of PCOS selected and evaluated 10 RCTs comparing clinical, hormonal and metabolic results [31]. TZDs were superior to metformin in reducing serum levels of free testosterone ($p = 0.03$) and dehydroepiandrosterone sulfate ($p = 0.002$) after 3 months of treatment. Decreases in triglyceride levels were more pronounced with metformin after 6 months ($p < 0.0001$). Decreases in BMI were greater with metformin treatment as assessed at 3 and 6 months ($p < 0.00001$). There were no significant between-group differences concerning improvements in ovulation, pregnancy rate, menstrual patterns or insulin sensitivity, or changes in serum levels of androstenedione, LH, FSH, total and HDL cholesterol, or insulin. Unfortunately, significant between-study heterogeneity was detected for several variables assessed. The findings from this meta-analysis do not indicate that metformin may be superior to TZDs for the treatment of PCOS or vice versa. The conclusion was that large-scale, well-designed, randomized, controlled trials are needed to further address this issue.

PCOS and Severe Insulin Resistance: A Target for Thiazolidinediones?

Insulin resistance commonly occurs in PCOS, particularly in the context of obesity. In some cases, however, insulin resistance is severe and is produced by a single genetic defect. These mutations also affect canonical insulin signaling. The underlying genetic defect can be inferred with some confidence from the characteristic syndrome features associated with the most severe impairment of insulin receptor function (Donohue syndrome and Rabson-Mendenhall syndrome) or from the pattern of fat loss in partial lipodystrophies [32]. However, severe insulin resistance most commonly manifests as a common form of PCOS associated with acanthosis nigricans and sometimes impaired glucose tolerance or T2D, dyslipidemia and hypertension, but without clinical features which permit reliable identification of these genetically determined forms of PCOS. In these forms, the degree of hyperinsulinemia is critical in guiding the diagnosis. However, there are no suggested criteria for the suspicion of severe insulin resistance in the event of partial β-cell decompensation and/or BMI >30. In these settings, clinical history, features such as acanthosis nigricans, and, perhaps, the lack of response to more widely used insulin sensitizers (such as metformin) assume particular importance [33].

To our knowledge, two forms of PCOS secondary to genetically determined severe insulin resistance are candidates for treatment with TZDs: (a) PCOS secondary to familial partial lipodystrophy 2 (FPLD2), and (b) PCOS secondary to familial partial lipodystrophy 3 (FPLD3). FPLD2, or Dunningan type, is produced by a lamin A/C (LMNA) gene mutation. This partial lipodystrophy usually becomes apparent during puberty and predominantly affects the limbs and gluteal fat depots with varying trunk involvement but with normal or excess fat on the face and neck and in the labia majora. Metabolic abnormalities range from asymptomatic impaired glucose tolerance and mild dyslipidemia to severe insulin resistance with T2D and severe dyslipidemia complicated by eruptive xanthomata and pancreatitis. Non-alcoholic fatty liver disease (NAFLD) and non-alcoholic steatohepatitis (NASH) are also common complications. Hypertension and accelerated atherosclerotic vascular disease have been reported in some patients. FPLD3 is produced by a PPARγ mutation. This is another partial lipodystrophy characterized by a paucity of limb and gluteal fat. It differs from FPLD2 in that abdominal fat is generally preserved and facial fat is often normal. In this case too, the lipodystrophy becomes clinically discernible during puberty in girls. Affected individuals usually manifest all the features of the metabolic syndrome including hypertension. Indeed, early-onset hypertension discriminates FPLD3 from FPLD2. NAFLD/NASH is almost universal, and some patients manifest severe hypertriglyceridemia. In support of what is mentioned above about the selective response to TZDs of these forms of PCOS is a case report [34] in which two sisters who presented with hyperandrogenism and menstrual disorders in the context of PCOS were subsequently found to be severely insulin resistant. Both sisters were found to be heterozygous for the R482Q mutation in the LMNA gene, and therefore to be affected by PCOS secondary to FPLD2. The introduction of pioglitazone (30 mg/day) after 2–3 years of uninterrupted therapy with metformin without any clinical and biochemical response resulted in progressive amelioration of insulin resistance, hyperinsulinemia, and hyperandrogenemia, an improvement of menses, with restoration of the eumenorrheic pattern, and a complete remission of the framework of ultrasound polycystic ovarian morphology.

Conclusions

Insulin resistance is a common feature of women with PCOS, particularly in the presence of obesity. Although the molecular mechanisms of insulin action are still not fully elucidated, it is quite clear that, in different ways, they involve not only classic insulin-sensitive tissues (liver, adipose tissue and muscles), but also the ovaries, where an altered insulin signaling pathway has been detected. Insulin resistance is in turn associated with compensatory hyperinsulinemia, which plays an important role in determining androgen excess production rates. According to the need, therapeutic options include lifestyle management (particularly in the presence of obesity), insulin sensitizers (metformin and TZDs), and antiandrogens, alone or in combination. Unfortunately, most of these treatments are not standardized, and recent consensus statements have focused on the treatment of anovulation and infertility rather than hyperandrogenism and metabolic abnormalities. In addition, the use of insulin sensitizers should be standardized, with particular attention to the specific phenotype and predictors of responsiveness. For example, there are very few studies performed in obese PCOS women with metformin combined with a lifestyle interventional program, which should by contrast be pursued by more intensive clinical research enthusiasm, as formerly demonstrated in the field of T2D. In fact, available data clearly indicate that lifestyle intervention and metformin may have an undisputed efficacy in the treatment of chronic anovulation and infertility in most PCOS patients, also in the preparation of assisted reproduction technologies. The use of TZDs as insulin-sensitizing agents seems to be particularly effective in PCOS women with severe insulin-resistant states, most of which probably depend on genetic mutations or polymorphisms of genes involved in the regulation of the insulin signaling pathway.

References

1. Ehrmann DA: Polycystic ovary syndrome. N Engl J Med 2005;352:1223.
2. Dunaif A: Insulin resistance and the polycystic ovary syndrome: mechanisms and implications for pathogenesis. Endocr Rev 1997;18:774.
3. Poretsky L, Cataldo NA, Rosenwaks Z, Giudice LC: The insulin-related ovarian regulatory system in health and disease. Endocr Rev 1999;20:535.
4. Palomba S, Falbo A, Zullo F, Orio F Jr: Evidence-based and potential benefits of metformin in the polycystic ovary syndrome: a comprehensive review. Endocr Rev 2009;30:1.
5. Diamanti-Kandarakis E: Metformin: an old medication of new fashion: evolving new molecular mechanisms and clinical implications in polycystic ovary syndrome. Eur J Endocrinol 2010;162:193.
6. Dunaif A: Drug insight: insulin-sensitizing drugs in the treatment of polycystic ovary syndrome – a reappraisal. Nat Clin Pract Endocrinol Metab 2008; 4:272.
7. Pasquali R, Gambineri A: Targeting insulin sensitivity in the treatment of polycystic ovary syndrome. Expert Opin Ther Targets 2009;13:1205.

8 Viollet B, Guigas B, Sanz Garcia N, Leclerc J, Foretz M, Andreelli F: Cellular and molecular mechanisms of metformin: an overview. Clin Sci 2012;122:253.
9 Zhou G, Myers L, Li Y, Chen Y, Shen X, Fenyk-Melody J, Wu M, Ventre J, Doebber T, Fuji N: Role of AMP-activated protein kinase in mechanism of metformin action. J Clin Invest 2001;108:1167.
10 Lord JM, Flight IH, Norman RJ: Metformin in polycystic ovary syndrome: systematic review and meta-analysis. BMJ 2003;327:951.
11 Kashyap S, Wells GA, Rosenwaks Z: Insulin-sensitizing agents as primary therapy for patients with polycystic ovary syndrome. Hum Reprod 2004; 19:2474.
12 Tang T, Lord JM, Norman RJ, Yasmin E, Balen AH: Insulin-sensitising drugs (metformin, rosiglitazone, pioglitazone, D-chiro-inositol) for women with polycystic ovary syndrome, oligo amenorrhoea and subfertility. Cochrane Database Syst Rev CD003053;2010.
13 Karimzadeh MA, Javedani M: An assessment of lifestyle modification versus medical treatment with clomiphene citrate, metformin, and clomiphene citrate-metformin in patients with polycystic ovary syndrome. Fertil Steril 2010;94:216.
14 Johnson NP, Stewart AW, Falkiner J, et al: PCOSMIC: a Multi-Centre Randomized Trial in Women with Polycystic Ovary Syndrome Evaluating Metformin for Infertility with Clomiphene. Hum Reprod 2010; 25:1675.
15 Palomba S, Pasquali R, Orio F Jr, Nestler JE: Clomiphene citrate, metformin or both as first-step approach in treating anovulatory infertility in patients with polycystic ovary syndrome (PCOS): a systematic review of head-to-head randomized controlled studies and meta-analysis. Clin Endocrinol (Oxf) 2009;70:311.
16 Moran LJ, Pasquali R, Teede HJ, Hoeger KM, Norman RJ: Treatment of obesity in polycystic ovary syndrome: a position statement of the Androgen Excess and Polycystic Ovary Syndrome Society. Fertil Steril 2009;92:1966–82.
17 Nathan DM, Buse JB, Mayer BD, Ferrannini E, Holman RR, Sherwin R, Zinman B: Medical management of hyperglycemia in type 2 diabetes: a consensus algorithm for the initiation and adjustment of therapy. A Consensus Statement of the American Diabetes Association and the European Association for the Study of Diabetes. Diabetes Care 2008;32:1.
18 Graham GG, Punt J, Arora M, Day RO, Doogue MP, Duong JK, Furlong TJ, Greenfield JR, Greenup LC, Kirkpatrick CM, Ray JE, Timmins P, Williams KM: Clinical pharmacokinetics of metformin. Clin Pharmacokinet 2011;50:81.
19 Moll E, Van Der Veen F, Van Wely M: The Role of Metformin in Polycystic Ovary Syndrome: a Systematic Review. Hum Reprod Update 2007; 13: 527.
20 Legro RS, Barnhart HX, Schlaff WD, et al: Reproductive Medicine Network. Ovulatory response to treatment of polycystic ovary syndrome is associated with a polymorphism in the STK11 gene. J Clin Endocrinol Metab 2008;93:792.
21 Shu Y, Sheardown SA, Brown C, Owen RP, Zhang S, Castro RA, Ianculescu AG, Yue L, Lo JC, Burchard EG: Effect of genetic variation in the organic cation transporter 1 (OCT1) on metformin action. J Clin Invest 2007;117:1422.
22 Zhou K, Donnelly LA, Kimber CH, Donnan PT, Doney AS, Leese G, Hattersley AT, McCarthy MI, Morris AD, Palmer CN, Pearson ER: Reduced-function SLC22A1 polymorphisms encoding organic cation transporter 1 and glycemic response to metformin: a GoDARTS Study. Diabetes 2009; 58:1434.
23 Gambineri A, Tomassoni F, Ibarra Gasparini D, di Rocco A, Mantovani V, Pagotto U, Altieri P, Sanna S, Fulghesu AM, Pasquali R: Organic cation transporter 1 polymorphism predict the metabolic response to metformin in women with polycystic ovary syndrome. J Clin Endocrinol Metab 2010;95: E204–E208.
24 Willson TM, Lambert MH, Kliewer SA: Peroxisome proliferator-activated receptor gamma and metabolic disease. Annu Rev Biochem 2001;70:341.
25 Kahn CR, Flier JS, Bar RS, Archer JA, Gorden P, Martin MM, Roth J: The syndromes of insulin resistance and acanthosis nigricans. Insulin-receptor disorders in man. N Engl J Med 1976;294:739.
26 Froment P, Touraine P: Thiazolidinediones and fertility in polycystic ovary syndrome (PCOS). PPAR Res 2006;2006:73986.
27 Brettenthaler N, De Geyter C, Huber PR, Keller U: Effect of insulin sensitizer pioglitazone on insulin resistance, hyperandrogenism, and ovulatory dysfunction in women with polycystic ovary syndrome. J Clin Endocrinol Metab 2004;89:3835.
28 Rautio K, Tapanainen JS, Ruokonen A, Morin-Papunen LC: Endocrine and metabolic effects of rosiglitazone in overweight women with PCOS: a randomized placebo-controlled study. Hum Reprod 2006;21:1400.
29 Aroda VR, Ciaraldi TP, Burke P, Mudaliar S, Clopton P, Phillips S, Chang RJ, Henry RR: Metabolic and hormonal changes induced by pioglitazone in polycystic ovary syndrome: a randomized, placebo-controlled clinical trial. J Clin Endocrinol Metab 2009;94:469.

30 Yki-Jarvinen H: Thiazolidinediones. N Engl J Med 2004;351:1106.
31 Li XJ, Yu YX, Liu CQ, Zhang W, Zhang HJ, Yan B, Wang LY, Yang SY, Zhang SH: Metformin vs thiazolidinediones for treatment of clinical, hormonal and metabolic characteristics of polycystic ovary syndrome: a meta-analysis. Clin Endocrinol (Oxf) 2011;74:332.
32 Kahn CR, Flier JS, Bar RS, Archer JA, Gorden P, Martin MM, Roth J: The syndromes of insulin resistance and acanthosis nigricans. Insulin-receptor disorders in man. N Engl J Med 1976;294:739.
33 Savage DB, Semple RK, Chatterjee VK, Wales JK, Ross RJ, O'Rahilly S: A clinical approach to severe insulin resistance. Endocr Dev 2007;11:122.
34 Gambineri A, Semple RK, Forlani G, Genghini S, Grassi I, Hyden CSS, Pagotto U, O'Rahilly S, Pasquali R: Monogenic polycystic ovary syndrome due to a mutation in the lamin A/C gene is sensitive to thiazolidinediones but not to metformin. Eur J Endocrinol 2008;159:347.

Renato Pasquali, MD
Division of Endocrinology, Department of Clinical Medicine
S. Orsola-Malpighi Hospital, University Alma Mater Studiorum
Via Massarenti 9
IT–40138 Bologna (Italy)
Tel. +39 0 51 6364147, E-Mail renato.pasquali@unibo.it

Macut D, Pfeifer M, Yildiz BO, Diamanti-Kandarakis E (eds): Polycystic Ovary Syndrome. Novel Insights into Causes and Therapy. Front Horm Res. Basel, Karger, 2013, vol 40, pp 103–114

Hirsutism – From Diagnosis to Use of Antiandrogens

Kursad Unluhizarci · Zuleyha Karaca · Fahrettin Kelestimur

Department of Endocrinology, Erciyes University Medical School, Kayseri, Turkey

Abstract

Hirsutism affects 5–8% of the whole female population. It results either from an increase in circulating androgen concentrations, an increase in the sensitivity of the pilosebaceous unit to normal androgen concentrations or a combination of these factors. Polycystic ovary syndrome is the underlying cause in the vast majority of patients with hirsutism; however, it should be kept in mind that it can only be diagnosed after exclusion of some other diseases such as non-classical congenital adrenal hyperplasia, Cushing's syndrome, hyperprolactinemia and acromegaly. The most important purpose for investigation is to identify those women with pathologies that can be potentially life threatening either due to their systemic effects or malignant potential. Specific causes of hirsutism such as Cushing's syndrome and adrenal/ovarian tumors should be treated by surgical excision of the tumor. In the other patients, pharmacological approach is the mainstay of the therapy. Antiandrogens can be competitive antagonists of the androgen receptor (spironolactone, cyproterone acetate, flutamide) or inhibitors of 5-α reductase, which decrease the conversion of testosterone to the more potent androgen 5-α dihydrotestosterone (finasteride). Antiandrogens should be used only after ensuring safe nonhormonal contraception to avoid fetal male pseudohermaphroditism in case of unplanned pregnancy.

Hirsutism is the main hyperandrogenic symptom defined as an excess of body hair in androgen-sensitive skin regions of women, and results either from an increase in circulating androgen concentrations, an increase in the sensitivity of the pilosebaceous unit (PSU) to normal androgen concentrations or a combination of these factors [1]. It negatively influences psychological well-being of young women. Hirsutism affects 5–8% of the whole female population of the reproductive age, and it may be associated with underlying endocrine and metabolic disturbances or may be the initial manifestation of potentially life-threatening disease such as androgen secreting tumors [2]. Although polycystic ovary syndrome (PCOS) is responsible for most of the cases, a number of other pathologic entities can present with hirsutism either alone or associated with other symptoms/signs of hyperandrogenism and/or other symptoms/signs

Table 1. Causes of hirsutism

Common causes
PCOS
Idiopathic hirsutism
NCAH
Idiopathic hyperandrogenemia
Rare causes
Adrenal/ovarian tumors
Cushing's syndrome
Acromegaly
Hyperprolactinemia
Thyroid dysfunction
HAIR-AN syndrome
Hyperthecosis
Glucocorticoid resistance syndrome
Drugs

suggestive of a specific disease. The management of hirsutism involves a range of diagnostic and therapeutic issues, and it is therefore essential to identify the underlying cause of hirsutism (table 1).

Pathophysiology of Hirsutism

There are approximately 5 million hair follicles covering the human body with nearly 100,000 located on the scalp. Hair follicles form exclusively during fetal development and very few new hair follicles are formed after birth. Hair follicles decrease in number after the age of 40 years. PSU number is genetically determined and it is approximately equal in men and women. The PSU is a highly dynamic system that changes throughout the lifespan. Hair grows in asynchronous cycles comprising three phases. An active growing phase (anagen), followed by an involutional stage (catagen), in which the hair stops growing and the hair bud shrinks, and finally, the telogen phase in which the hair is resting, and then sheds, as new hair displaces it [3]. Hirsutism is not due to an increase in number or concentration of hair follicles but rather a change in the quantity of the hair fiber, such as size, degree of pigmentation and the length of the produced hair. Sex steroids and a number of local and systemic factors can act directly and indirectly on dermal papilla to regulate hair growth. Various hormones, growth factors and cytokines have been observed to affect hair growth.

Androgens, mainly testosterone and dihydrotestosterone (DHT), are the most important hormones determining the type and distribution of hairs over the human body. The majority of circulating testosterone is tightly bound to a specific transport glycoprotein, sex hormone-binging globulin (SHBG). Only free testosterone is biologically available to enter target tissues. Accordingly, circulating SHBG can modulate the bioavailability of testosterone and contribute to the clinical manifestations of androgen excess. The production rate of SHBG by the liver is increased by estrogens and thyroid hormone and decreased by androgens and insulin. Under the influence of androgens, hair follicles that are producing vellus type hairs can be transformed to terminal hairs. Additionally, androgens prolong the anagen phase of body hairs, while shortening the anagen phase of scalp hairs which eventually leads to hirsutism and alopecia [3, 4]. Androgens affect scalp follicles differently to those elsewhere. On the scalp, androgens miniaturize follicles leading to patterned balding or androgenetic alopecia. These paradoxical effects on hairs from various regions of the body are caused by different paracrine factors. Androgen excess at the scalp induces TGF-β and results in cyclical miniaturization of the entire follicle. On the beard area, androgens induce IGF-2, which results in cyclical enlargement of the entire hair follicle. Hair transplantation experiments indicate that this paradoxical effect is due to genetically determined regional specificity of hair follicle androgen response [4].

In addition to the effects of circulating androgens on the growth of sexual hair, human sebaceous glands and hair follicles are equipped with all the necessary enzymes for biosynthesis and metabolism of androgens [5]. Therefore, circulating androgen levels may not reflect local androgen concentrations at the PSU. It is well known that the severity of hirsutism does not correlate well with circulating androgen concentrations explaining some women with hirsutism may have normal serum androgen levels.

The major androgens in the serum of normal cycling women are DHEAS, DHEA, androstenedione, testosterone and DHT. Apart from testosterone and DHT, other androgens do not bind to the androgen receptor and may be considered as prohormones. Circulating testosterone in women originates mostly (50%) from peripheral conversion of other androgenic steroids, the rest coming in equal parts from the ovaries and the adrenal glands. The effect of androgens on the development of terminal hairs is mediated through 5-α reductase (5α-R) activity which is the product of the function of two distinct isoenzymes, type 1 and type 2 5α-R, distributed widely throughout the body [6]. Both types of 5α-R can be localized to the outer root sheath of the hair follicle. The activity of local 5α-R determines the production of DHT and consequently, the effect of androgens on hair follicles.

In the PSU, DHT stimulates increased sebum production, the differentiation of the hair follicle from vellus to terminal hairs and the prolongation of the anagen phase resulting in longer and thicker hairs. Polymorphisms in the androgen receptor gene also influence the activity of the receptor. However, there are inconsistent data regarding the role of these polymorphisms in hirsutism. Because androgens stimulate the growth of terminal hair by prolonging its anagen phase, the clinical effects of androgen excess and of its amelioration necessarily takes months to be apparent to both the patient and physician.

Clinical Evaluation and Differential Diagnosis of Hirsutism

A detailed history including medication, menstrual and reproductive history, the onset and the progression of hirsutism, acne and hair loss should be obtained. In addition to regular physical examination, it is essential to evaluate the amount and the distribution of the excessive hair while taking into consideration specific variations mainly due to differences in the genetic background of the various populations affected by hirsutism [7, 8].

There are a number of methods for the evaluation of hirsutism in women, including objective and subjective ones. Objective methods include photographic evaluations, weighing of plucked hair or microscopic measurements. Those methods are complex, costly and inconvenient for daily practice. Subjective methods refer to visually scoring terminal body and facial hair growth in specified areas. Although several visually scoring methods have been described, a modified Ferriman-Gallwey scoring system [9] has now become the most preferred method for the evaluation and treatment of hirsutism. In this scoring system, hair growth at different body sites (upper lip, chin/face, chest, upper and lower back, upper and lower abdomen, arm, thigh) is evaluated. In each area, absence of terminal hairs (score 0) to extensive terminal hair growth (score 4) is assigned. Scoring hirsutism requires considerable experience and although a score of 8 or more is accepted as indicative of hirsutism, it has been suggested that the cutoff value should be ideally established for each population.

Hirsutism must be differentiated from hypertrichosis which refers to vellus type hair growth all over the body which does not reflect hyperandrogenism. Vellus hairs are short, soft, fine and usually non-pigmented. Terminal hairs are long, coarse, medullated and pigmented. Hypertrichosis is characterized by increased hair growth located in non-androgen-dependent area, and may be encountered in anorexia nervosa, hypothyroidism, administration of drugs such as cyclosporin, phenytoin and diazoxide, or it may be a paraneoplastic manifestation, a condition called hypertrichosis lanuginosa [10]. However, some patients exhibit both, hirsutism and hypertrichosis; in these cases, clinical expression of hirsutism is more severe than its actual hirsutism score.

Depending on the severity of androgenization, signs of virilization, an uncommon clinical finding of androgen excess, may also be seen. This condition is usually associated with remarkably elevated serum androgen levels and is characterized by androgenetic alopecia, clitoromegaly, deepening of the voice, increased muscle mass, and decreased/atrophic breast size.

The degree and distribution of androgen-dependent signs do not indicate any specific cause of hyperandrogenism. Furthermore, the severity of hirsutism does not correlate well with the magnitude of androgen excess. Therefore, establishing the etiology of hirsutism in all patients irrespective of its severity is essential (fig. 1). The most common hyperandrogenic disorder is PCOS affecting approximately 65–85% of women with androgen excess [7, 8]. The diagnostic criteria of PCOS have changed

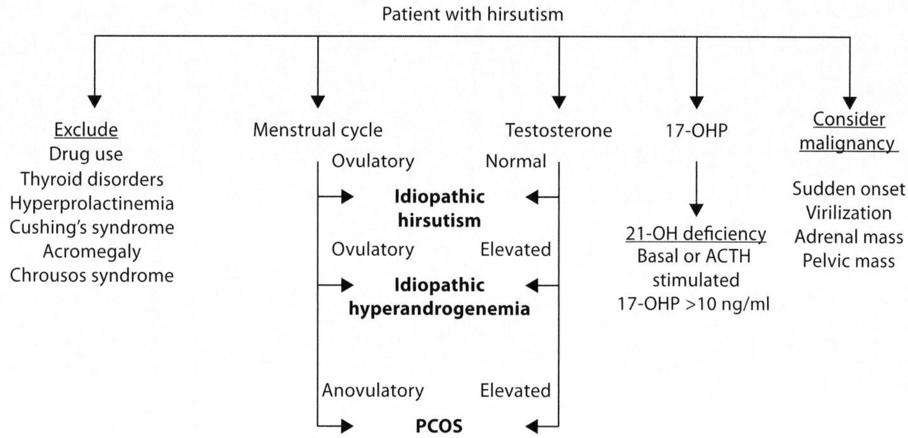

Fig. 1. Evaluation of patients with hirsutism. Adapted from Unluhizarci et al. [7].

over time, and as understanding of the molecular and genetic aspects of the disorder increases, the definition will be expanded. Currently, PCOS is diagnosed in patients with hyperandrogenism (hirsutism and/or hyperandrogenemia) and ovarian dysfunction (oligoanovulation and/or polycystic ovaries) and exclusion of other androgen excess or related disorders such as 21-hydroxylase (21-OH)-deficient non-classic adrenal hyperplasia (NCAH), androgen-secreting tumors, Cushing's syndrome, hyperandrogenemia-insulin resistance-acanthosis nigricans (HAIR-AN) syndrome, thyroid dysfunction and hyperprolactinemia [11]. Since PCOS is frequently associated with insulin resistance, abdominal obesity and/or acanthosis nigricans are frequent findings. Approximately 3% of hyperandrogenic women suffer from HAIR-AN syndrome that is considered as a distinct group, but most authors include these patients within the PCOS spectrum.

In approximately 1–8% of the women with hirsutism, the underlying cause of the disease is NCAH which shares many features with PCOS. Although 21-OH deficiency represents the most common form of NCAH, it has been previously reported that NCAH due to 11-β hydroxylase deficiency may be more common in some populations [12–14]. 21-OH deficiency is diagnosed by the measurement of a basal 17-hydroxyprogesterone (17-OHP) level. If the 17-OHP level is over 2 ng/ml (6 nmol/l), the patient should undergo an ACTH stimulation test. An ACTH-stimulated 17-OHP concentration greater than 10 ng/ml (30 nmol/l) was considered as the hormonal criteria for NCAH due to 21-OH deficiency. The diagnosis should be confirmed by molecular biology studies if possible.

Some hirsute patients do not have evidence of detectable androgen excess or endocrine imbalance, as in women with 'idiopathic hirsutism'. Idiopathic hirsutism can be diagnosed in hirsute patients who have normal serum androgen levels and regular menstrual cycles. Depending on ethnicity and the geographic area, idiopathic hirsutism constitutes 5–17% of the patients with hirsutism [2, 7].

A number of patients have hyperandrogenemia with normal ovarian morphology and regular cycles. These patients also exhibit similar hormonal features to PCOS subjects and their condition is called idiopathic hyperandrogenemia [2, 8]. This group of patients may have functional ovarian and/or adrenal hyperandrogenism.

Androgen-secreting tumors are relatively rare, and they are one of the most important issues in the differential diagnosis of hirsutism. These tumors usually arise from the ovaries or the adrenal glands. Although malignant tumors are associated with higher serum androgen concentrations, there is no clear cutoff level of androgen concentrations for the differential diagnosis of benign versus malignant etiologies. A rapidly progressive onset of hyperandrogenism, particularly in postmenopausal women and/or development of frank virilization suggests an androgen-secreting tumor arising either from the ovaries or the adrenal glands [15]. Androgen-secreting adrenal tumors, mostly carcinomas are usually associated with the development of Cushingoid features and can be diagnosed as a typically large (>6 cm) mass on ultrasound or adrenal computerized tomography. Greater production of adrenal androgens, including DHEAS, has been shown in patients with carcinoma than in those with adenoma [16].

Finally, some drugs may also cause hirsutism, e.g. danazol, valproic acid (which is an important anticonvulsant drug that raises serum testosterone levels), and anabolic and androgenic steroids.

Laboratory Evaluation of Hirsutism

After obtaining a detailed medical history and performing physical examination, basal hormonal (mainly androgens) and ultrasonographic examination of the ovaries and the adrenal glands is a useful screening procedure, but not obligatory. If the symptoms suggest the presence of a neoplasm with negative ultrasonographic imaging, computerized tomography of the adrenal glands or the ovaries should be obtained. A correct etiological diagnosis is essential in order to exclude life-threatening conditions such as androgen-secreting tumors or the life-long consequences of some disorders associated with hirsutism such as PCOS and NCAH. Although hirsutism is an important marker of androgen excess, the severity of hirsutism does not correlate with serum androgen levels. Additionally, hirsutism may also be influenced by other hormonal variables including insulin resistance and hyperinsulinemia. Thus, certain tests must be conducted to ascertain properly the etiology of hirsutism.

However, there is no universal consensus regarding the least required tests for the differential diagnosis of hirsutism. Hormonal status of the patient should be established during the follicular phase of menstrual cycle. The initial laboratory

Table 2. Suggested laboratory investigations in women with hirsutism

Laboratory investigation	Contribution
FSH-LH-estradiol	Evaluation of gonadal axis
Testosterone	Establishment of androgen excess
SHBG	Indirect measure of androgen excess Contributes to calculate FAI
Free androgen index (FAI)	Extensively used as a measure of androgen excess
17-OHP	Screening of NCAH due to 21-OH deficiency
ACTH test (cortisol and 17-OHP)	Hormonal diagnosis of NCAH due to 21-OH deficiency
Ultrasonography	Evaluation of ovaries and the adrenal glands

investigations include testosterone, free androgen index (calculated by measuring SHBG and total testosterone levels), androstenedione, thyroid function tests, prolactin and 17-OHP level. At least one determination of serum androgen levels should be obtained in patients with hirsutism before starting any treatment that might interfere with such measurements.

During the last decade, a serious debate has been raised regarding the value of commercial direct immunoassays used for serum androgen measurements. Of all circulating androgens, assessment of free testosterone levels are much more sensitive than the measurement of total testosterone for the diagnosis of hyperandrogenic disorders. Free testosterone measurements ideally require equilibrium dialysis techniques and should not rely on direct analog radioimmunoassays. Several societies have questioned the use of these assays for the measurement of serum androgen levels in children and women, and suggest more sensitive methods that couple extraction by liquid chromatography with tandem mass spectrometry. However, recently Legro et al. [17] demonstrated that there is still utility and potentially cost savings in the measure of total testosterone by direct RIA in hyperandrogenic women. The diagnostic performance of measuring serum total testosterone may be enhanced by the concomitant measurement of SHBG, permitting the estimation of free testosterone levels that have a fairly good correlation with free testosterone as measured by equilibrium dialysis methods. Suggested investigations in women with hirsutism are given in table 2.

Principles of Treatment in Women with Hirsutism

The main goals of the management of hirsutism are ameliorating hirsutism, to prevent and/or treat the possible metabolic abnormalities associated and, if possible, to treat the underlying cause. Obesity has a negative impact on the efficacy of treatment for hirsutism; thus, appropriate lifestyle advice is necessary for a successful treatment program.

Table 3. Antiandrogens used in the treatment of hirsutism

Drug	Usual dose	Indication	Disadvantage
Spironolactone	100 mg/day	Any form of hirsutism	Menstrual irregularities Postural hypotension Dizziness
CPA	2 mg in combination with ethinylestradiol or 12.5–100 mg/day alone for 10 days in each cycle	Particularly in PCOS	Hepatotoxicity (in high doses)
Finasteride	2.5–5 mg/day	Any form of hirsutism	No major adverse event
Flutamide	62.5–250 mg/day	Any form of hirsutism	Hepatotoxicity

Specific causes of hirsutism such as Cushing's syndrome and adrenal/ovarian tumors should be treated by surgical excision of the tumor. In other patients, pharmacological approach is the mainstay of therapy. Pharmacological treatment of hirsutism is directed at slowing the growth of new hair, and the options are antiandrogens, combined oral contraceptive pill (OCP) with or without antiandrogen agents, gonadotropin-releasing hormone agonists and rarely insulin sensitizers. Antiandrogens can be competitive antagonists of the androgen receptor (spironolactone, cyproterone acetate – CPA, flutamide) or inhibitors of 5-α-R, which decrease the conversion of testosterone to the more potent androgen 5-α DHT (finasteride). Another antiandrogen, bicatulamide, had been used in a limited number of patients, and there are not enough data regarding its effect on hirsutism. A general overview of antiandrogens used in the treatment of hirsutism is given in table 3.

Patients should be informed about the type and the duration of the therapy. Generally, more than 6 months are necessary in order to evaluate the success of the medical therapy. The treatment of hirsutism involves the prevention of excessive androgen secretion and/or the blockade of androgens. The selection of the drug/drugs depends on the severity of the hirsutism score, associated conditions such as menstrual irregularities and any contraindication to possible therapeutic agent. Patients should be aware that most of the drugs used in the management of hirsutism are contraindicated in women desiring pregnancy, and simultaneous treatment of infertility and hirsutism is difficult. Thus, in hirsute patients in whom OCPs are contraindicated, antiandrogens should be used only after ensuring safe nonhormonal contraception to avoid fetal male pseudohermaphroditism in case of unplanned pregnancy.

PCOS is the most common cause of hirsutism. Nearly 70% of women with PCOS are obese, and they should be encouraged to lose weight. OCPs are the most common drugs used for the suppression of ovarian androgen production [1, 18]. Among OCPs, those containing a progestin with low androgenic activity may be preferable. Several new progestins have been synthesized in the past decade, including drospirenone, nestorone and trimegestone. OCPs can be used either alone or in combination with antiandrogens, and the details of OCPs will not be discussed since they are reviewed in another chapter.

Antiandrogen treatment is one of the main therapeutic approaches in the treatment of hirsutism. The great majority of patients with hirsutism are prescribed antiandrogens as the first-line treatment or they are added later. Only few patients use other therapeutic options alone, but antiandrogen drugs. Particularly during the last 20 years, a lot of studies on the effectiveness of antiandrogen therapy in the treatment of hirsutism have been published. Therefore, we have got more experience concerning the administration of antiandrogens in hirsute women. Antiandrogen agent may be used alone, combined with another antiandrogen agent or may be combined with an OCP. Despite remarkable progression in the field of hirsutism treatment, still no perfect antiandrogen drug is available. The agents that we choose for the treatment of hirsutism should be effective, safe and cheap.

CPA is a steroidal antiandrogen derived from 17-OHP. It is one of the most widely used drugs in the management of hirsutism and works by various mechanisms. It is both an antiandrogen and a progestagen which binds to the DHT receptor in the cytoplasm in the hair follicle preventing its translocation into the nucleus to cause an androgenic effect. In addition to this receptor activity, it inhibits 5α-R activity reducing DHT production, and also inhibits the production of gonadotropins. The reduced gonadotropin levels in turn reduce steroidogenesis. The recommended dose of CPA for premenopausal women is 50 or 100 mg/day for 10 days per cycle. Studies comparing various dosages of CPA did not demonstrate any noticeable differences in decreasing the hirsutism scores between high and low dosages. In accordance, the most commonly used form is 2 mg CPA combined with 35 μg ethinyl estradiol [19]. CPA may cause headache, weight gain, breast tenderness, nausea, loss of libido, edema, hepatotoxicity, fatigue, mood changes. If the patient who is on CPA wishes pregnancy, CPA should be stopped at least two cycles before the pregnancy to avoid the risk of feminizing a male fetus.

Peripheral blockade of androgen actions at the skin is an effective method in the treatment of hirsutism. Finasteride, which is a 5α-R inhibitor blocks the conversion of testosterone to the more potent DHT. It does not bind to the androgen receptor but binds to the 5α-R enzyme and interferes with its action. 5α-R has two isoenzymes including 5α-R type 2 which is found predominantly in genital skin and the prostate in the male and 5α-R type 1 which is found in the scalp, pubic skin and non-sex skin. Finasteride is more effective against isoenzyme 5α-R type 2 than type 1, but the specificity for these two isoenzymes is incomplete. Finasteride has been used in the treatment of hirsutism with various doses [20]. In those studies, the authors report that low-dose (2.5 mg/day) finasteride therapy is as effective as high (5 mg/day) dose therapy with similar side-effect profile. Finasteride has teratogenic potential and should be used with effective contraception.

An aldosterone antagonist spironolactone is also an androgen receptor antagonist and the most commonly used antiandrogen drug. Spironolactone competes with androgens for the binding to androgen receptor and inhibits the interaction of DHT with its intracellular receptor, increases the metabolic clearance of testosterone, and inhibits androgen production. It is generally effective in doses between 50 and 200 mg. The side effects of spironolactone include breast tenderness and enlarged breasts, transient diuresis, dizziness, headache, hyperkalemia (it is not important in patients with normal kidney function), gastrointestinal discomfort, nausea, allergic reactions, fatigue, somnolence, vertigo, polyuria and polydipsia, particularly in the first days of treatment. Spironolactone is commonly used in a dose of 100 mg/day and rarely 200 mg/day. Spironolactone may lead to polymenorrhea, and its frequency has been reported as 50–60%. Spironolactone used as a single agent is as effective as CPA combined with estradiol for long-term treatment of patients with hirsutism [21]. It has been shown that a combination of two antiandrogens (spironolactone-finasteride) with different mechanisms of action may be used in women with hirsutism [22]. Although spironolactone and finasteride are classified as antiandrogen drugs, there are important differences in their mechanisms of action. It has been shown that after one year of treatment, combination of these agents resulted in significant percent change (51.3%) in hirsutism score from baseline in comparison to spironolactone alone (36.6%) without increased side effects [22]. Surprisingly, polymenorrhea was seen less frequently in patients who used the combination therapy.

A new progestin derived from 17α-spironolactone, drospirenone, shares progesterone's antiandrogenic and antimineralocorticoid properties with no androgenic, estrogenic, glucocorticoid or antiglucocorticoid activity. Drospirenone has been demonstrated to display antiandrogenic activity at the peripheral level by competitive binding to the androgen receptor that is intrinsic to its molecular structure. The blockade of androgen receptors in the skin represents an additional mechanism when combined with ethinyl estradiol. In addition to blocking androgen receptors, drospirenone inhibits ovarian androgen production [23].

Flutamide is a non-steroidal antiandrogen. It has been shown that low doses (62.5–250 mg/day) of flutamide are very effective in the treatment of hirsutism [24]. Although in several studies the effects of finasteride and flutamide have been clearly shown, combination of finasteride (5 mg/day) plus flutamide (125 mg/day) was not more effective than flutamide alone [25]. This result was unexpected since such a combination therapy with different (or at least theoretically, complementary) mechanisms of action might result in better improvement than either drug used alone. Thus, it should be emphasized that not all combination therapies for hirsutism work well. In comparison to spironolactone and finasteride, the latter combination has a lower safety profile and serious liver toxicities have been reported, particularly at high doses. During flutamide therapy, liver function tests should be monitored regularly.

Among women with hirsutism, metabolic abnormalities such as hypertension, glucose intolerance and/or insulin resistance and lipid abnormalities have consistently been shown in women with PCOS. Metformin is an alternative therapy for hirsutism in women with PCOS who have other indications for metformin use. Metformin is not as effective as antiandrogens in the management of hirsutism. But it may be combined with an antiandrogen agent to increase the effectiveness of the treatment [26].

Treatment of hirsutism depends on the underlying cause. The most common causes of hirsutism are PCOS, idiopathic hirsutism and idiopathic hyperandrogenemia. The type of antiandrogen agent and duration of therapy should be individualized.

References

1 Azziz R: The evaluation and management of hirsutism. Obstet Gynecol 2003;101:995.
2 Carmina E, Rosato F, Janni A, Rizzo M, Longo RA: Relative prevalence of different androgen excess disorders in 950 women referred because of clinical hyperandrogenism. J Clin Endocrinol Metab 2006; 91:2.
3 Uno H: Biology of hair growth. Semin Reprod Endocrinol 1986;4:131.
4 Rashidi M, Sinclair R: Diagnosis and treatments of hirsutism: where are we? Expert Rev Dermatol 2011;6:423.
5 Thiboutot D, Jabara S, McAllister JM, Sivarajah A, Gilliland K, Cong Z, Clawson G: Human skin is a steroidogenic tissue: steroidogenic enzymes and cofactors are expressed in epidermis, normal sebocytes, and an immortalized sebocyte cell line (SEB-I). J Invest Dermatol 2003;120:905.
6 Thigpen AE, Silver RI, Guilleyard JM, Casey ML, McConnell JD, Russell DW: Tissue distribution and ontogeny of steroid 5-alpha reductase isoenzyme expression. J Clin Invest 1993;92:903.
7 Unluhizarci K, Kaltsas G, Kelestimur F: Non polycystic ovary syndrome-related endocrine disorders associated with hirsutism. Eur J Clin Invest 2012; 42:86.
8 Unluhizarci K, Gokce C, Atmaca H, Bayram F, Kelestimur F: A detailed investigation of hirsutism in a Turkish population: idiopathic hyperandrogenemia as a perplexing issue. Exp Clin Endocrinol Diabetes 2004;112:504.
9 Hatch R, Rosenfield RL, Kim MH, Tredway D: Hirsutism: implications, etiology, and management. Am J Obstet Gynecol 1981;140:815.
10 Rittmaster RS: Hirsutism. Lancet 1997;349:191.
11 Azziz R, Carmina E, Dewailly D, Diamanti-Kandarakis E, Escobar-Morreale E, Futterweit W, Janssen OE, Legro RS, Norman RJ, Taylor AE, Witchel SF: The Androgen Excess and Polycystic Ovary Syndrome Society criteria for the polycystic ovary syndrome: the complete task force report. Fertil Steril 2009;91:456.
12 Unluhizarci K, Kula M, Dundar M, Tanriverdi F, Israel S, Colak R, Dokmetas HS, Atmaca H, Bahceci M, Balci MK, Comlekci A, Bilen H, Akarsu E, Erem C, Kelestimur F: The prevalence of non-classic adrenal hyperplasia among Turkish women with hyperandrogenism. Gynecol Endocrinol 2010;26:139.
13 Young J, Tardy V, de la Perriere AB, Bachelot A, Morel Y: Detection and management of late-onset 21-hydroxylase deficiency in women with hyperandrogenism. Ann Endocrinol 2010;71:14.
14 Kelestimur F, Sahin Y, Ayata D, Tutus A: The prevalence of non-classic adrenal hyperplasia due to 11β-hydroxylase deficiency among hirsute women in a Turkish population. Clin Endocrinol 1996; 45:381.
15 Kaltsas GA, Isidori AM, Kola BP, Skelly RH, Chew SL, Jenkins PJ, Monson JP, Grossman AB, Beser GM: The value of low-dose dexamethasone supression test in the differential diagnosis of hyperandrogenism in women. J Clin Endocrinol Metab 2003; 88:2634.
16 Midorikawa S, Hashimoto S, Kuriki M, Katoh K, Watanabe T, Sasano H, Nishikawa T: A patient with preclinical Cushing's syndrome and excessive DHEA-S secretion having unilateral adrenal carcinoma and contralateral adenoma. Endocr J 1999; 46:59.
17 Legro RS, Schlaff WD, Diamond MP, et al: Total testosterone assays in women with polycystic ovary syndrome: precision and correlation with hirsutism. J Clin Endocrinol Metab 2010;95:5305.
18 Azziz R, Gay F: The treatment of hyperandrogenism with oral contraceptives. Semin Reprod Endocrinol 1989;7:246.
19 Franks S, Layton A, Glasier A: Cyproterone acetate/ethinyl estradiol for acne and hirsutism: time to revise prescribing policy. Hum Reprod 2008;23:231.
20 Bayram F, Muderris II, Guven M, Kelestimur F: Comparison of high-dose finasteride (5 mg/day) versus low-dose finasteride (2.5 mg/day) in the treatment of hirsutism. Eur J Endocrinol 2002; 147:467.

21 Spritzer PM, Lisboa KO, Mottiello S, Lhullier F: Spironolactone as a single agent for long-term therapy of hirsute patients. Clin Endocrinol 2000; 52:587.
22 Kelestimur F, Everest E, Unluhizarci K, Bayram F, Sahin Y: Comparison between spironolactone and spironolactone plus finasteride in the treatment of hirsutism. Eur J Endocrinol 2004;150:351.
23 Guido M, Romualdi D, Giuliani M Suriano R, Selvaggi L, Apa R, Lanzone A: Drospirenone for the treatment of hirsute women with polycystic ovary syndrome: a clinical, endocrinological, metabolic pilot study. J Clin Endocrinol Metab 2004;89:2817.
24 Muderris II, Bayram F, Guven M: Treatment of hirsutism with lowest dose flutamide (62.5 mg/day). Gynecol Endocrinol 2000;14:38.
25 Unluhizarci K, Ozel D, Tanriverdi F, Karaca Z, Kelestimur F: A comparison between finasteride, flutamide, and finasteride plus flutamide combination in the treatment of hirsutism. J Endocrinol Invest 2009;32:37.
26 Diamanti-Kandarakis E, Economou F, Palimeri S, Christakou C: Metformin in polycystic ovary syndrome. Ann N Y Acad Sci 2010;1205:192.

Fahrettin Kelestimur, MD
Department of Endocrinology, Erciyes University Medical School
TR–38039 Kayseri (Turkey)
Tel. + 90 352 437 49 37, E-Mail fktimur@erciyes.edu.tr

Macut D, Pfeifer M, Yildiz BO, Diamanti-Kandarakis E (eds): Polycystic Ovary Syndrome. Novel Insights into Causes and Therapy. Front Horm Res. Basel, Karger, 2013, vol 40, pp 115–127

Combined Oral Contraceptives in Polycystic Ovary Syndrome – Indications and Cautions

Gurkan Bozdag[a] · Bulent Okan Yildiz[b]

[a]Department of Obstetrics and Gynecology, and [b]Endocrinology and Metabolism Unit, Department of Internal Medicine, Hacettepe University School of Medicine, Ankara, Turkey

Abstract

Combined oral contraceptive pills (OCPs) have been used in women with polycystic ovary syndrome (PCOS) for the treatment of menstrual disorders, acne and hirsutism. Despite years of their use and broad clinical experience, there are still ongoing doubts concerning their implications for the cardiovascular system and carbohydrate metabolism both in the general population and women with PCOS. In the general population, the risk of venous thromboembolism is reported to be increased. However, arterial thrombotic events seem to require concomitant risk factors to appear during administration of OCPs. In terms of carbohydrate metabolism, available data do not consistently suggest an increased risk of impaired glucose tolerance (IGT) or conversion of IGT to type 2 diabetes mellitus, in spite of some subtle fluctuations in glucose and insulin levels. In subgroup analyses of epidemiological studies in the general population, there is no finding indicating an increased risk of cardiovascular disease and related mortality in premenopausal women with PCOS. There is no significant alteration in carbohydrate and lipid metabolism after use of OCP in PCOS either. The absence of further cardiometabolic risk with OCP use in PCOS might suggest some unproven preventive alterations in this patient population.

Combined oral contraceptive pills (OCPs) are the most frequently used type of contraception in the general population with a failure rate of 0.3% per year in the presence of perfect use [1]. Besides contraception, OCPs are used for the treatment of menstrual irregular bleeding, severe dysmenorrhea, hirsutism, acne, dysfunctional uterine bleeding, endometriosis and even to schedule the cycles in in vitro fertilization. They can be either 'monophasic' with constant dosage of estrogen and progestagens or 'triphasic' with changing dosage of progestagens, which brings lower dosage of sex steroids in the beginning of the cycle.

Polycystic ovary syndrome (PCOS) is a common endocrine disorder associated with a high risk of menstrual disorders and hirsutism. Therefore, OCPs are commonly prescribed in clinical practice for the management of symptoms. However, while deciding on an OCP, a general concern arises due to high risk of metabolic syndrome in PCOS and well-known effects of such drugs on cardiovascular and carbohydrate/lipid metabolism.

In the current report, we first discuss the usage of OCP and related risk in healthy women, and then we extrapolate these findings to the patients with PCOS and review the limited data on that issue.

Oral Contraceptive Pills: Are They All the Same?

While almost all OCPs contain ethinyl estradiol (EE), only a few of them include mestranol in which 3-methyl ether is adjoined to EE. A total dose of >50 and <50 μg EE is called high- and low-dose pills, respectively. With time, the total dose of EE has gradually decreased. Nowadays, most of the pills contain ≤35 μg of EE, which is assumed to decrease the complications attributed to the high dose of estradiol.

The progestagen component of the OCP may present various chemical structures, clinical effects and metabolic risks. The classification of progestagens within the OCP in the literature is also confusing. Up to now, there have been four generations of progestagens that have been announced within the OCPs. The first generation includes norethindrone or an agent that is converted to norethindrone (norethindrone acetate, ethynodiol diacetate) after metabolization, and they are called the 'estrane' family. Second and third generations are called the 'gonane' family. While the second generation consists of levonorgestrel and norgestrel which bring high progestational and androgenic effects, the third generation includes norgestimate, and desogestrel that reveal high progestational performance but minimized androgenic effects and estrogenic activity. The fourth generation is typical with its antiandrogenic effect. A member of this group is drospirenone which is derived from 17α-spironolactone instead of 19-nortestosterone and has slight antiandrogenic effects. Other progestins that have antiandrogenic effects in the same group are cyproterone acetate and dienogest. While cyproterone acetate has the highest antiandrogenic effect, dienogest and drospirenone have 40 and 30% potency of cyproterone, respectively [2]. They block androgen receptors in the skin, reduce the activity of 5α-reductase in hair follicles, and diminish ovarian and adrenal androgen production. The use of antiandrogens in PCOS is reviewed in detail in the chapter by Unluhizarci et al. [pp. 103–114].

It is clear that all the OCPs are not the same, and they might present diversity related to their type of progestins rather than the dosage of estradiol. They have various effects not only on sex steroid synthesis, but also on the hematologic system which is called 'total estrogenicity' and will be discussed below.

Administration

Before prescribing any kind of OCP, a careful medical history should be taken, and blood pressure measurement has to be done. Although some physicians advocate performing breast exams, cervical pap smear and screening for sexually transmitted diseases, most professional societies including the American College of Obstetricians and Gynecologists, the World Health Organization, and the Royal College of Obstetricians and Gynecologists agree that these procedures are not necessary before the first prescription for OCPs. After 3 months, a revisit might be scheduled to check the blood pressure and OCP should be continued if the patient is comfortable with the drug. An annual visit might be required to control for further compliance and side effects.

Although OCPs can be started at any time during the cycle, if it is done during the first 5 days of the menstrual bleeding, then there is no need for further method of contraception in the current cycle.

Contraindications

There are certain conditions in which either the theoretical or proven risks usually outweigh the advantages or represent an unacceptable health risk of using the OCP [3]:

- Previous or current thromboembolic event
- Up to 1 month of postpartum period in women who are breastfeeding
- Up to 21 days of postpartum period in women who are not breastfeeding
- Advanced age (≥35 years) in the presence of smoking
- Women who underwent a jejunoileal bypass due to decreased absorption
- Multiple risk factors for arterial cardiovascular disease, CVD (such as older age, smoking, diabetes, and hypertension)
- Hypertension with systolic blood pressure ≥160 mm Hg or diastolic ≥100 mm Hg
- Known thrombophilia, including antiphospholipid syndrome
- Active cancer (metastatic, on therapy, or within 6 months after clinical remission), excluding non-melanoma skin cancer
- Prolonged immobilization
- Known thrombogenic mutations (e.g. factor V Leiden, prothrombin mutation, protein S, protein C, and antithrombin deficiencies). Still, routine screening is not appropriate because of the rarity of the conditions and the high cost of screening
- Current and history of ischemic heart disease
- History of cerebrovascular accident
- Complicated valvular heart disease (pulmonary hypertension, risk for atrial fibrillation, history of subacute bacterial endocarditis)
- History of peripartum cardiomyopathy

Table 1. OCP use and cardiometabolic risk in the general population and in PCOS

	Reference	Remarks
General population		
VTE in general population	2	0.8/10,000 women/year
OCP use and VTE		3–4/10,000 women/year
VTE in pregnancy		6–10/10,000 women/year
Current OCP use and MI	11	OR: 2.48 (1.91–1.35)
	12	OR: 1.84 (1.38–2.44)
Current OCP and ischemic stroke	12	OR: 2.12 (1.56–2.86)
OCP and carbohydrate metabolism	16	Increased insulin secretion of 60–90% Increased insulin half-life of 28% Higher plasma glucose level of 18–40%
	19	No increased risk of DM
PCOS		
OCP and CVD	27, 28	Increase in HDL only
	29	Increase in TG and HDL
OCP and carbohydrate metabolism	29	No change in fasting insulin, glucose disposal rate or FG/I Increase in TG and HDL

VTE = Venous thromboembolism; DM = diabetes mellitus; FG/I = fasting glucose/insulin; TG = triglyceride.

- Systemic lupus erythematosus, if antiphospholipid antibodies are positive or unknown
- Migraine (at any age with aura or without aura ≥35 years)
- Current or past breast disease for <5 years

Oral Contraceptive Pill Use and Related Cardiovascular Risk in General Population

The use of OCP is associated with venous thrombosis [2]. Whereas the risk of venous thromboembolic event (VTE) is 0.8/10,000 women-year in the general population, this risk increases to 3–4/10,000 in women taking OCP. However, in the presence of pregnancy, the risk of VTE is 6–10/10,000 and goes to approximately 50/10,000 in the puerperal period. Therefore, the baseline risk in young women is low and the absolute risk is smaller than the actual risk associated with pregnancy [2]. On the other hand, the worldwide usage of OCPs is 93 million per year, and after a rough estimation, we may assume that 20,000 women will suffer from VTE related to OCPs every year (table 1).

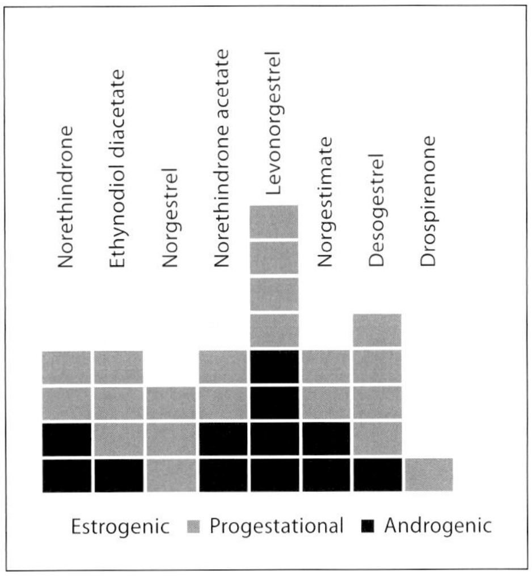

Fig. 1. Comparison of progestins according to their androgenic, estrogenic and progestational effects.

The first reports of VTE associated with OCPs were published in 1960s [4]. Biochemically, while fibrinogen, prothrombin, factors VII, VIII, and X are increasing, factor V seems to be decreasing in the coagulation system with OCP use. On the other hand, within the anticoagulation system, activated protein C (APC) resistance significantly increases, and tissue factor pathway inhibitor, antithrombin, prothrombin C inhibitor and α-1 antitrypsin levels all decrease [5]. The fluctuations in the fibrinolysis do not seem to be responsible for the increased risk of cardiovascular complications [6]. Mainly, increased resistance of APC is assumed to be responsible for the complications of OCPs [7]. Furthermore, monitoring the changes in APC resistance after any hormonal contraception can be used to predict the possible risk of VTE with the treatment [5]. This estimation can also be done by analyzing the increase in sex hormone-binding globulin (SHBG) level after the treatment, when the pretreatment levels are referred [5]. Of interest, the highest increment in SHBG of 300–400% is caused by cyproterone acetate [5]. The 2nd and 3th generations of progestins bring a rise of 200–300% in SHBG levels compared with baseline values [5]. On the other hand, levonorgestrel brings a rise of just 50%. The fluctuations in APC resistance are similar to those observed in SHBG levels. These findings indicate an increased incidence of VTE in users of OCPs with later generation of progestins. Concordantly, as a clinical finding, when compared with the 2nd generation, the risk of VTE increases 1.5- to 2-fold and 2- to 4-fold in the 3rd and 4th generations of progestins, respectively [8]. Once again, the term 'total estrogenicity' is crucial for the risk of VTE, and reflects the characteristics of progestin rather than the dosage of estrogen that it includes. The comparisons of progestins regarding their estrogenic, progestational and androgenic effects are depicted in figure 1. Of note, most of the venous thromboembolic complications occur during the first three months of treatment. Past users have not been noticed to be at risk.

The data on arterial thrombosis such as cerebrovascular or cardiac event with OCP are less conclusive. Strokes in young women are rare with an incidence of 3/100,000 women/year [9]. These rates are increased in combined hormonal contraception users with the already established risk factors such as smoking (2- to 4-fold), hypertension (7- to 8-fold), and adverse lipids profile (10- to 11-fold) [10]. However, in otherwise healthy young women (non-smokers without hypertension), the attributable risk is low because the baseline risk of ischemic stroke is already rare in that population. As a matter of fact, some studies failed to show any risk of thromboembolic stroke in OCP users when compared with non-users. Similar to venous thromboembolism, high-dose estrogen pills might be associated with higher risk than low-dose pills, but do not differ according to 2nd or 3rd generation progestin that is used. The usage of OCP in women having migraine with aura doubles the risk of stroke, and that is why it is recommended to select another type of contraception in such patients.

According to a meta-analysis done in 2003 reviewing 19 case-control and 4 cohort studies, current OCP use yields an adjusted OR of 2.48 (CI 1.91–1.35) for myocardial infarction (MI) when compared with never-users [11]. The analysis was significant both for smokers and non-smokers and for young (<35 years) and older (≥35 years) users. The risk of MI for past OCP users was not significantly different from that of never-users, with an overall OR of 1.15 (0.98–1.35) [11]. In another meta-analysis [12] including 15 studies, the summary risk estimates associated with current use of low-dose OCPs were 1.84 (1.38–2.44) for MI and 2.12 (1.56–2.86) for ischemic stroke [12] (table 1). Whereas second generation OCPs were associated with a significantly increased risk of both MI and ischemic stroke events, only ischemic stroke was relevant with third-generation OCPs [12]. Of interest, four independent studies reported in that meta-analysis argued on the risk of cardiovascular events with past use of low-dose OCPs as compared with never use. The authors noticed a significant reduction of risk for both MI and ischemic stroke [13] outcomes in past users when compared with current users. Similarly, in the Women's Ischemia Syndrome Evaluation (WISE) study [14], in which 672 postmenopausal women were enrolled undergoing coronary angiography for suspected myocardial ischemia, the authors reported that, past OCP use was associated with a lower mean coronary artery disease severity index score compared with non-prior users, despite age adjustment.

Prescribing OCPs in the presence of smoking is an important issue for the physicians in their clinical practice. A consensus panel reviewing the issue of oral contraceptives in women over 35 who smoke suggested that OCPs should not be given to those who smoke more than 15 cigarettes per day, but they can be considered in women who smoke fewer than 15 cigarettes per day, since the risks of pregnancy in this age group are greater than the risks associated with OCP use. On the other hand, for younger women, the benefits of OCPs appear to outweigh the risks, even among heavy smokers.

Overall, for clinical practice we can assume that use of OCP is associated with the risk of VTE, and this risk might further increase according to the type of progestin used, particularly in the first months of the treatment. Secondly, the cardiovascular risk is noticed to be increased in current OCP users, but not in the past ones. Thirdly, the association with ischemic stroke, if it exists, is small in healthy women. Classic risk factors such as hypertension, migraine with aura, hypertension and diabetes mellitus accompanying end organ damage might exaggerate the baseline risks and deserve further attention.

Oral Contraceptive Pill Use and Carbohydrate Metabolism in General Population

The effect of OCPs on carbohydrate metabolism depends on the dose of estrogen, type of progestin and demographic features of the women. When several types of OCPs were tested, the greatest effect on carbohydrate metabolism was obtained by levonorgestrel-containing combinations, followed by desogestrel and norethindrone [2]. While levonorgestrel combinations with EE increased second-phase pancreatic insulin secretion by 60–90% without any effect on the half-life of insulin, desogestrel combination increased the insulin half-life by 28% without any decrease in insulin secretion [15]. The same group also noticed that, overall, users had 43–61% higher plasma glucose levels, 12–40% higher insulin resistance (IR) and 18–40% higher C peptide response compared to non-users. In contrast, cross-sectional data including 3,000 women in the Third National Health and Nutrition Examination Survey revealed that fasting glucose, insulin and C peptide levels were similar between users, never-users or past users. Another prospective observational study (CARDIA) investigating the risk of diabetes in young women also supported those findings for current users [16].

The largest study prospectively investigating OCP use and subsequent incidence of diabetes was reported in 1992 by Rimm et al. [17]. The authors followed 115,117 women for 12 years and concluded that, even though current users of OCP did not have an increased risk of diabetes, past users had a relative risk of 1.10 (1.01–1.21) [17]. However, in a follow-up study [18] by the same group of investigators, (n = 98,590 women, 4 years' follow-up), neither current nor past users were found to be at increased risk of diabetes after adjusting for demographic features, smoking, dyslipidemia and hypertension.

To sum up, although subtle biochemical alterations on carbohydrate metabolism might be observed among OCP users, solid data supporting an increased risk of diabetes with such a treatment are still lacking.

The Need for Oral Contraceptive Pills in PCOS

PCOS is a systemic disorder characterized by hyperandrogenism, ovulatory dysfunction and/or polycystic ovaries on ultrasound. Related to its symptoms, OCPs

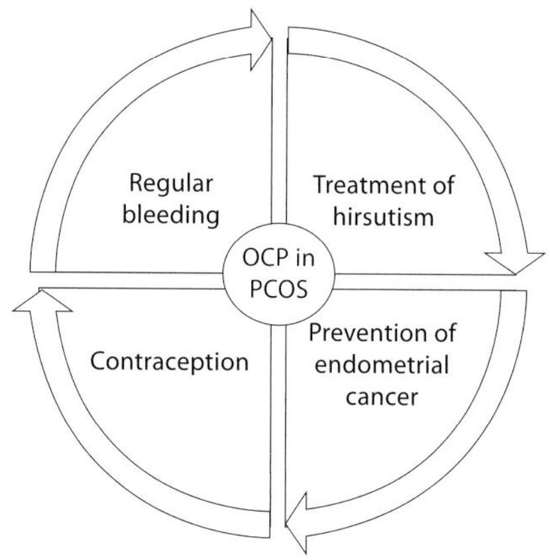

Fig. 2. Rationality of OCP use in PCOS.

have a wide range of usage in PCOS (fig. 2). However, potential deleterious effects of OCPs on hemostasis and insulin sensitivity might induce a suspicion of exaggerating the cardiometabolic risk of the syndrome that has already been shown in several studies.

Menstrual irregularity constitutes another issue related to the syndrome. Approximately 5% of cases with endometrial cancer occur in women aged 40 years and younger in whom chronic anovulation is a strong risk factor. Obesity, diabetes and IR are other risk factors for endometrial cancer often occurring in PCOS. That finding suggests in every patient who does not ovulate and does not want to have children, endometrium should be protected either with progestagen or OCP. The preventive effect of OCP on endometrial cancer among general population has been widely investigated and could be extrapolated to patients with PCOS.

The therapeutic effect of OCPs on hyperandrogenism includes more than one mechanism of action: (1) suppression of androgen production in the ovary by inhibiting pituitary secretion of LH for as much as 70%, (2) induction of SHBG synthesis in the liver after 3–4 weeks and consequent decrease in free testosterone levels to 50% of the baseline, (3) a slight decrease in adrenal androgen production, and (4) direct antiandrogenic effect of a progestin component of OCPs, such as cyproterone acetate.

According to either subjective or objective scales, OCP effectively reduces hirsutism and acne in women with PCOS. This improvement is noted to be 60–100% after at least 6 months of treatment. Often, OCPs are prescribed in combination with an antiandrogen to block androgen action at the hair follicles. The most cited progestin that is used along with an OCP is spironolactone, a mineralocorticoid and androgen receptor blocker [19]. Destruction of the hair follicles by epilation should be recommended as an adjuvant treatment in order to increase effectiveness, particularly after completing the 6th month of the hormonal suppression.

Diabetes, obesity, IR, dyslipidemia, hypertension and impaired fibrinolysis are significant risk factors for CVD which can be noted more frequently in women with PCOS than in the general population [2, 19]. The PCOS population has a higher prevalence of metabolic syndrome with an OR of 2.20 (1.36–3.56) compared to healthy women even in BMI-matched studies [20], and the prevalence rates are reported between 15 and 44% [21].

Regarding the serum markers of CVD, the PCOS population has elevated high sensitivity C-reactive protein and homocysteine levels compared to age- and BMI-matched controls. A recent meta-analysis of 16 studies with a total of 1,186 women showed that PCOS women had lower adiponectin levels than control women [22], which in turn has been associated with progression to type 2 diabetes [23]. Increased carotid artery intima media thickness [24] and coronary heart calcification [25] are clinical findings of the syndrome which can be attributed to the syndrome per se or metabolic complications related with it. However, according to the available epidemiological studies, an increased risk of CVD and related morbidity and mortality in premenopausal women with PCOS has not been proven yet [2].

According to the limited number of observational studies that assess risk factors related to CVD, after 3 years of treatment with EE and cyproterone acetate, an increase in triglyceride and a relative decrease in high-density lipoprotein (HDL) were noted [26]. In another observational study reporting a survey of up to 10 years [27], total cholesterol and triglycerides did not change in either group, but HDL cholesterol increased only in OCP users [27]. According to a recent meta-analysis of observational studies [28], even though total cholesterol ($p = 0.36$) or LDL ($p = 0.14$) did not change after OCP use, a significant increase in HDL was observed after treatment ($p = 0.004$). However, when subgroup analysis was performed, there was a significant association ($p = 0.01$) with a BMI of 30 or higher, whereas those studies with a BMI of 30 or less did not show a significant association between OCP use and HDL. OCP use was also significantly associated with an increase in triglycerides ($p = 0.004$), especially in studies when OCP was prescribed for 6 months or longer. There was no significant difference across mean BMI subgroups.

Of interest, waist circumference, the waist-to-hip and the waist-to-thigh ratios decreased significantly only in the OCP users. Neither of the studies was able to evaluate the MI or stroke.

From the findings of studies evaluating OCP and CVD in the general population, as mentioned above, we can assume that when OCP in women with PCOS is stopped, there is no ongoing risk for the remaining years of life. In addition, due to the lack of evidence that presents increased risk of MI or stroke among individuals with PCOS, one may hypothesize that current OCP use may not exaggerate baseline risk further, because most women would probably be taking an OCP, due to hirsutism or menstrual irregularity. However, it is noteworthy to recall that there is no study directly evaluating the influence of OCP on cardiovascular mortality and morbidity in patients with PCOS.

Oral Contraceptive Pill Use and Future Risk of Diabetes in PCOS

IR is assumed to exist in the majority of women with PCOS. As a clinical sign of that assumption, impaired glucose tolerance (IGT) and type 2 diabetes are reported to be increased in women with PCOS when compared with general population. In a study of 122 obese women with PCOS, 35% had IGT and type 2 diabetes by age 40 [29]. Of interest, in a second study of 71 women with PCOS, the annual conversion rate from normal glucose tolerance to IGT was reported to be as high as 17% [30]. In a series of 394 women [31], none of the 52 women with a BMI less than 27.0 had the metabolic syndrome, whereas those in the top BMI quartile were 13.7 times more likely (5.7–33.0) to have the metabolic syndrome compared with those in the lowest quartile. In addition, 38% of those with the metabolic syndrome had IGT compared with 19% without the metabolic syndrome ($p < 0.001$). According to a recent meta-analysis including a total of 35 trials for final analysis, women with PCOS had increased prevalence of IGT and type 2 diabetes even in BMI-matched studies. The respective odds ratios were 4.43 (4.06–4.82) for IGT and 4.00 (1.97–8.10) for diabetes [20]. A recent long-term (mean follow-up 16.9 years) prospective study of a large cohort of women with PCOS ($n = 255$), followed from youth to middle age, evaluated both the incidence and potential predictors of diabetes in PCOS [32]. Whereas the age-standardized prevalence of diabetes at the end of follow-up was 39.3%, the general Italian female population of a similar age was 5.8%. The likelihood of developing type 2 diabetes increased significantly when BMI, fasting glucose and glucose area under the curve at baseline increased, whereas the risk of diabetes decreased when SHBG levels at follow-up increased [32].

As mentioned above, available studies suggest that OCP use might increase the IR and C-peptide production in the general population, even though there are no data indicating that there is a high risk for conversion to apparent diabetes. However, one may hypothesize that there might be a further risk when compared with general population among women with PCOS due to underlying IR. Of note, the hyperandrogenic subgroup is reported to have a higher risk of IR, and is a likely candidate for prescribing OCP for a necessary period of time.

According to a recent meta-analysis including 35 studies [28], OCPs with various types of progestagen use in PCOS was not associated with a change in fasting glucose ($p = 0.69$), fasting insulin ($p = 0.07$) or fasting glucose to insulin ratio ($p = 0.41$). Neither HOMA-IR ($p = 0.45$) nor euglycemic hyperinsulinemic clamp – glucose disposal rate ($p = 0.96$) showed any association with OCP use.

Another therapeutic option for insulin-resistant women with PCOS under consideration for OCP might be insulin sensitizers such as metformin. A Cochrane review included six trials, four of which compared metformin versus OCP (suggested to state the OCP formulations used; n = 104) and two of which compared OCP (EE/CPA) combined with metformin versus OCP alone (n = 70) [33]. Of note, there were no trials assessing cardiovascular outcome. Metformin, in comparison with the OCP, was more effective in reducing fasting insulin (weighted mean difference = –3.46 (–5.39 to –1.52) and not increasing fasting triglyceride (weighted mean difference = –0.48, (–0.86 to –0.09) levels. Limited data demonstrated no evidence of a difference between the two therapies in effect on reducing fasting glucose or total cholesterol levels and severe adverse events [33]. Another systematic review [34] retrieved seven studies comparing EE/CPA with metformin with a duration of 3–12 months and revealed no difference for the prevalence of IGT, fasting glucose or diabetes. Only triglycerides showed a significant difference between groups (weighted mean difference = 0.48 (0.09–0.86), being higher in the EE/CPA group.

As a result, there is no documented risk of conversion to IGT or type 2 diabetes by giving OCP to patients with PCOS.

Conclusion

Combined OCPs are not only used with the aim of contraception but also for the treatment of menstrual abnormalities, hirsutism and acne in clinical practice. The type of progestin and dosage of estrogen might influence side effects and complication rates such as venous thromboembolism in the general population. However, arterial thrombosis including MI and cerebrovascular events and the relation to the usage of OCP is less clear due to the low rate of incidence. Of note, the fluctuations in carbohydrate and lipid metabolism are not severe enough to suppose significant risks in the long term.

Women with PCOS are candidates for the use of OCP for these indications: menstrual dysfunction, hirsutism and endometrial protection. However, there are some confusing points that are discussed above: (1) women with PCOS have already increased baseline prevalence of metabolic syndrome and some biochemical findings associated with CVD risk; (2) women with PCOS may require use of OCP for a long period of time; (3) antiandrogen with contraception properties, cyproterane acetate, is one of the agents that have the highest potency for VTE. Related to those issues, one may hypothesize accelerated risk of cardiometabolic complications in PCOS with the use of OCPs when compared with the general population. However, the lack of sufficient evidence might suggest unproven factor(s) in this condition that could balance with negative biochemical findings such as hyperinsulinemia, increased levels of homocysteine or high sensitivity C-reactive protein. Nevertheless, the long-term use of OCP might in part be responsible for the absence of increased cardiovascular morbidity in PCOS despite various alterations in surrogate risk markers that have been shown in many studies. As cited in the WISE study [14] and by Baillargeon et al. [12], the finding of fewer coronary artery disease and ischemic stroke cases in past OCP users compared with never-users also supports potential beneficial effect. That assumption is compatible with the finding in the general population that earlier initiation of hormone therapy might be associated with less angiographic coronary artery disease in women with natural menopause [35].

References

1 Speroff L, Darney PD: A Clinical Guide for Contraception, ed 3. Philadelphia, Lippincott Williams and Wilkins, 2001.

2 Yildiz BO: Oral contraceptives in polycystic ovary syndrome: risk-benefit assessment. Semin Reprod Med 2008;26:111–120.

3 Centers for Disease Control and Prevention: US Medical Eligibility Criteria for Contraceptive Use. Atlanta, Centers for Disease Control and Prevention, 2010.

4 Boyce J, Fawcett JW, Noall EW: Coronary thrombosis and Conovide. Lancet 1963;1:111.

5 Tchaikovski SN, Rosing J: Mechanisms of estrogen-induced venous thromboembolism. Thromb Res 2010;126:5–11.

6 Harris GM, Stendt CL, Vollenhoven BJ, Gan TE, Tipping PG: Decreased plasma tissue factor pathway inhibitor in women taking combined oral contraceptives. Am J Hematol 1999;60:175–180.

7 Rosing J, Tans G, Nicolaes GA, Thomassen MC, van Oerle R, van der Ploeg PM, Heijnen P, Hamulyak K, Hemker HC: Oral contraceptives and venous thrombosis: different sensitivities to activated protein C in women using second- and third-generation oral contraceptives. Br J Haematol 1997; 97:233–238.

8 van Hylckama Vlieg A, Helmerhorst FM, Vandenbroucke JP, Doggen CJ, Rosendaal FR: The venous thrombotic risk of oral contraceptives, effects of oestrogen dose and progestogen type: results of the MEGA case-control study. BMJ 2009; 339:b2921.

9 DeLoughery TG: Estrogen and thrombosis: controversies and common sense. Rev Endocr Metab Disord 2011;12:77–84.

10 Rosendaal FR, Van Hylckama Vlieg A, Tanis BC, Helmerhorst FM: Estrogens, progestogens and thrombosis. J Thromb Haemost 2003;1:1371–1380.

11 Khader YS, Rice J, John L, Abueita O: Oral contraceptives use and the risk of myocardial infarction: a meta-analysis. Contraception 2003;68:11–17.

12 Baillargeon JP, McClish DK, Essah PA, Nestler JE: Association between the current use of low-dose oral contraceptives and cardiovascular arterial disease: a meta-analysis. J Clin Endocrinol Metab 2005;90:3863–3870.

13 Schwartz SM, Siscovick DS, Longstreth WT Jr, Psaty BM, Beverly RK, Raghunathan TE, Lin D, Koepsell TD: Use of low-dose oral contraceptives and stroke in young women. Ann Intern Med 1997;127:596–603.

14 Merz CN, Johnson BD, Berga S, Braunstein G, Reis SE, Bittner V: Past oral contraceptive use and angiographic coronary artery disease in postmenopausal women: data from the National Heart, Lung, and Blood Institute-sponsored Women's Ischemia Syndrome Evaluation. Fertil Steril 2006; 85:1425–1431.

15 Sitruk-Ware R, Nath A: Metabolic effects of contraceptive steroids. Rev Endocr Metab Disord 2011;12: 63–75.

16 Kim C, Siscovick DS, Sidney S, Lewis CE, Kiefe CI, Koepsell TD: Oral contraceptive use and association with glucose, insulin, and diabetes in young adult women: the CARDIA Study. Coronary Artery Risk Development in Young Adults. Diabetes Care 2002;25:1027–1032.

17 Rimm EB, Manson JE, Stampfer MJ, Colditz GA, Willett WC, Rosner B, Hennekens CH, Speizer FE: Oral contraceptive use and the risk of type 2 (non-insulin-dependent) diabetes mellitus in a large prospective study of women. Diabetologia 1992;35: 967–972.

18 Chasan-Taber L, Willett WC, Stampfer MJ, Spiegelman D, Rosner BA, Hunter DJ, Colditz GA, Manson JE: Oral contraceptives and ovulatory causes of delayed fertility. Am J Epidemiol 1997;146: 258–265.

19 Fauser BC, Tarlatzis BC, Rebar RW, et al: Consensus on women's health aspects of polycystic ovary syndrome (PCOS): the Amsterdam ESHRE/ASRM-Sponsored 3rd PCOS Consensus Workshop Group. Fertil Steril 2012;97:28–38, e25.

20 Moran LJ, Misso ML, Wild RA, Norman RJ: Impaired glucose tolerance, type 2 diabetes and metabolic syndrome in polycystic ovary syndrome: a systematic review and meta-analysis. Hum Reprod Update 2010;16:347–363.
21 Mak W, Dokras A: Polycystic ovarian syndrome and the risk of cardiovascular disease and thrombosis. Semin Thromb Hemost 2009;35:613–620.
22 Orio F Jr, Palomba S, Cascella T, Tauchmanova L, Nardo LG, Di Biase S, Labella D, Russo T, Savastano S, Tolino A, Zullo F, Colao A, Lombardi G: Is plasminogen activator inhibitor-1 a cardiovascular risk factor in young women with polycystic ovary syndrome? Reprod Biomed Online 2004;9:505–510.
23 Jalovaara K, Santaniemi M, Timonen M, Jokelainen J, Kesaniemi YA, Ukkola O, Keinanen-Kiukaanniemi S, Rajala U: Low serum adiponectin level as a predictor of impaired glucose regulation and type 2 diabetes mellitus in a middle-aged Finnish population. Metabolism 2008;57:1130–1134.
24 Orio F, Palomba S, Colao A: Cardiovascular risk in women with polycystic ovary syndrome. Fertil Steril 2006;86(suppl 1):S20–S21.
25 Legro RS: Polycystic ovary syndrome and cardiovascular disease: a premature association? Endocr Rev 2003;24:302–312.
26 Falsetti L, Pasinetti E: Effects of long-term administration of an oral contraceptive containing ethinylestradiol and cyproterone acetate on lipid metabolism in women with polycystic ovary syndrome. Acta Obstet Gynecol Scand 1995;74:56–60.
27 Pasquali R, Gambineri A, Anconetani B, Vicennati V, Colitta D, Caramelli E, Casimirri F, Morselli-Labate AM: The natural history of the metabolic syndrome in young women with the polycystic ovary syndrome and the effect of long-term oestrogen-progestagen treatment. Clin Endocrinol (Oxf) 1999;50:517–527.
28 Halperin IJ, Kumar SS, Stroup DF, Laredo SE: The association between the combined oral contraceptive pill and insulin resistance, dysglycemia and dyslipidemia in women with polycystic ovary syndrome: a systematic review and meta-analysis of observational studies. Hum Reprod 2011;26:191–201.
29 Ehrmann DA, Barnes RB, Rosenfield RL, Cavaghan MK, Imperial J: Prevalence of impaired glucose tolerance and diabetes in women with polycystic ovary syndrome. Diabetes Care 1999;22:141–146.
30 Legro RS, Gnatuk CL, Kunselman AR, Dunaif A: Changes in glucose tolerance over time in women with polycystic ovary syndrome: a controlled study. J Clin Endocrinol Metab 2005;90:3236–3242.
31 Ehrmann DA, Liljenquist DR, Kasza K, Azziz R, Legro RS, Ghazzi MN: Prevalence and predictors of the metabolic syndrome in women with polycystic ovary syndrome. J Clin Endocrinol Metab 2006;91:48–53.
32 Gambineri A, Patton L, Altieri P, Pagotto U, Pizzi C, Manzoli L, Pasquali R: Polycystic ovary syndrome is a risk factor for type 2 diabetes: results from a long-term prospective study. Diabetes 2012, Epub ahead of print.
33 Costello MF, Shrestha B, Eden J, Johnson NP, Sjoblom P: Metformin versus oral contraceptive pill in polycystic ovary syndrome: a Cochrane review. Hum Reprod 2007;22:1200–1209.
34 Jing Z, Liang-Zhi X, Tai-Xiang W, Ying T, Yu-Jian J: The effects of Diane-35 and metformin in treatment of polycystic ovary syndrome: an updated systematic review. Gynecol Endocrinol 2008;24:590–600.
35 Shufelt CL, Johnson BD, Berga SL, Braunstein GD, Reis SE, Bittner V, Yang Y, Pepine CJ, Sharaf BL, Sopko G, Kelsey SF, Merz CN: Timing of hormone therapy, type of menopause, and coronary disease in women: data from the National Heart, Lung, and Blood Institute-sponsored Women's Ischemia Syndrome Evaluation. Menopause 2011;18:943–950.

Bulent Okan Yildiz, MD
Endocrinology and Metabolism Unit, Department of Internal Medicine
Hacettepe University School of Medicine
Sihhiye
TR–06100 Hacettepe, Ankara (Turkey)
Tel. +90 312 3051707, E-Mail yildizbo@yahoo.com

Macut D, Pfeifer M, Yildiz BO, Diamanti-Kandarakis E (eds): Polycystic Ovary Syndrome. Novel Insights into Causes and Therapy. Front Horm Res. Basel, Karger, 2013, vol 40, pp 128–141

Infertility Treatment in Polycystic Ovary Syndrome: Lifestyle Interventions, Medications and Surgery

Dimitrios Panidis[a] · Konstantinos Tziomalos[b] · Efstathios Papadakis[a] · Ilias Katsikis[a]

[a]Division of Endocrinology and Human Reproduction, Second Department of Obstetrics and Gynecology, Hippokration Hospital, Aristotle University of Thessaloniki, and [b]First Propedeutic Department of Internal Medicine, AHEPA Hospital, Aristotle University of Thessaloniki, Thessaloniki, Greece

Abstract

Management of patients with polycystic ovary syndrome (PCOS) who wish to become pregnant should include exclusion of other diseases in the woman and additional fertility disorders in the couple. Before the initiation of any pharmacological intervention, the importance of lifestyle modifications should be stressed, particularly weight loss, increased exercise, smoking cessation and reduced alcohol consumption. The pharmacological treatment of choice for the induction of ovulation and for achieving live birth is the combination of metformin and clomiphene citrate. If this combination is unsuccessful, second-line treatments include the administration of gonadotropins and laparoscopic ovarian drilling. Induction of ovulation using clomiphene or gonadotropins leads to single live birth in 72% of cases, whereas laparoscopic ovarian drilling leads to live birth in 50% of cases. In vitro fertilization represents third-line treatment. Finally, individualized interventions can be implemented for the induction of ovulation depending on the specific characteristics of patients with PCOS. These interventions might deviate from the above-designated order of treatments in specific subgroups of patients with PCOS.

Polycystic ovary syndrome (PCOS) is the commonest endocrine disorder in women of reproductive age and the most frequent cause of anovulating infertility in developed countries. Common clinical manifestations of PCOS include menstrual disorders, due to the anovulation, and androgen excess signs, including hirsutism, oily skin, acne and androgenic alopecia [1].

A principal characteristic of PCOS is insulin resistance (IR) [1]. Another important feature of the syndrome is obesity. Indeed, 38–88% of patients with PCOS are overweight or obese [2]. The majority of patients of PCOS, regardless of bodyweight,

Table 1. Definition of PCOS phenotypes based on 2003 Rotterdam criteria [5]

PCOS phenotype	Oligo- or anovulation	Biochemical hyperandrogenemia or clinical manifestations of hyperandrogenemia	Polycystic ovaries in transvaginal ultrasonography
1 – severe PCOS	+	+	+
2 – oligo- or anovulation and hyperandrogenemia	+	+	–
3 – ovulatory PCOS	–	+	+
4 – mild PCOS	+	–	+

Phenotypes 1 and 2 were also included in the 1990 NIH criteria [7].

manifest a type of IR that is intrinsic to the syndrome and has uncertain pathogenesis. Obese patients with PCOS additionally have obesity-related IR [3].

PCOS is associated with major metabolic disorders, which are potentially due to the characteristic type of IR that accompanies the syndrome [1]. Indeed, the incidence of type 2 diabetes mellitus (T2DM) in the US is 10 times higher in patients with PCOS compared with healthy women. In addition, 30–50% of obese women with PCOS develop impaired glucose tolerance or T2DM after the age of 30 years [4].

Up to now, three key signs have been proposed for the diagnosis of PCOS. These include chronic oligo- or anovulation, biochemical hyperandrogenemia or clinical manifestations of hyperandrogenemia and polycystic ovaries on ultrasound [5]. It should be emphasized that the diagnosis of PCOS mandates the exclusion of other well-known disorders that cause or mimic the manifestations of PCOS.

There are currently two main definitions of PCOS, which are the subject of intense debate [6]. According to the 1990 criteria of the National Institutes of Health, the diagnosis of PCOS requires the presence of chronic oligo- or anovulation and biochemical or clinical hyperandrogenemia [7]. On the other hand, the 2003 Rotterdam criteria of the ESHRE/ASRM-sponsored PCOS Consensus Workshop Group [5] require the presence of at least two of the following three characteristics for the diagnosis of PCOS: (a) chronic oligo- or anovulation, (b) biochemical or clinical hyperandrogenemia, and (c) polycystic ovaries on ultrasound. The addition of a third diagnostic criterion, namely the presence of polycystic ovaries on ultrasound, results in four different phenotypes of PCOS (table 1).

The Rotterdam definition created several problems with implications in the clinical diagnosis of PCOS and in the design of clinical studies [6]. The Androgen Excess and PCOS Society recently issued guidelines which recommend that PCOS should be primarily considered as a disorder of excess in androgen synthesis, activity or metabolism [8]. Therefore, ovulating patients with biochemical hyperandrogenemia or clinical manifestations of hyperandrogenemia and polycystic ovaries (phenotype 3; table 1) have a mild form of PCOS. On the other hand, regarding patients with chronic oligo- or anovulation and polycystic ovaries (phenotype 4; table 1), even though preliminary data suggest that they manifest subtle endocrine and metabolic disorders that resemble mild PCOS, their metabolic characteristics are currently considered too mild or not associated with increased risk for metabolic disorders that characterize patients with PCOS.

Causes of Infertility in Patients with PCOS

Infertility in patients with PCOS is due to oligo- or anovulation. PCOS is mainly a cause of oligo-ovulation rather than anovulation. From time to time, due to unknown reasons, a follicle becomes dominant and can escape from the inhibitory intraovarian effect and proceed to ovulation and formation of corpus luteum. Because of these random episodes of ovulation, fertility rates in patients with PCOS without treatment are not zero, even though they are lower than in healthy ovulating women. In addition, some patients with PCOS have regular ovulation (ovulatory PCOS, phenotype 3; table 1) and normal fertility despite the presence of biochemical hyperandrogenemia or clinical manifestations of hyperandrogenemia [9].

Five theories have been proposed for the explanation of anovulation in PCOS: (a) the theory of auto-inhibitory effect on the reservoir of available for selection follicles due to their excessive number [10], (b) the theory of the premature effect of LH on the granulosa cells of the available for selection follicles [11], (c) the theory of follicular unresponsiveness due to the presence of IR and compensatory hyperinsulinemia [12], (d) the theory of increased activity of catechol-o-methyltransferase in the granulose cells of the follicles [13], (e) the theory of oocyte abnormalities [14], and (f) the theory of elevated anti-müllerian hormone inducing follicular arrest by interacting negatively with follicle-stimulating hormone (FSH) [15].

Besides oligo- or anovulation, other factors also contribute to the infertility in patients with PCOS. It is well established that during the induction of multiple ovulation for in vitro fertilization (IVF), a large number of oocytes is retrieved from patients with PCOS. However, these oocytes are of poor quality, leading to low rates of fertilization, cleavage and implantation and higher miscarriage rates. The latter are not associated with higher rates of fetal aneuploidy. Other non-chromosomal factors are implicated in the increased miscarriage rates in patients with PCOS. The failure of oocyte maturation and fetal development in these patients are probably due to abnormal endocrine and paracrine factors, metabolic disorders and alterations in the intrauterine environment during folliculogenesis and follicular maturation. Therefore, a better understanding of the association between PCOS and the abnormal extra- and intraovarian factors and of the effects of the latter factors on the cross-talk between granulosa cells and the oocyte, the maturation of the oocyte and the embryonic development. This better understanding will improve clinical stimulation and fertility and increase live birth rates in patients with PCOS undergoing IVF [16].

A substantial proportion of patients with PCOS is obese [2] and has the metabolic syndrome [17]. These two disorders reduce considerably the functionality of the reproductive system. The precise pathophysiologic pathway through which obesity exerts its detrimental action is unclear. However, both animal and clinical studies suggest that obesity has adverse effects on all the levels of the hypothalamus-pituitary-ovary axis. Indeed, obesity affects ovulation, oocyte maturation, endometrial development, uterine responsiveness and fetal implantation and miscarriage. Accordingly, weight loss represents the treatment of choice in obese women with infertility [18–20].

Lifestyle Interventions

Lifestyle change programs, which emphasize behavior control and interventions of diet and exercise, have been shown to be very effective in improving the reproductive as well as the metabolic characteristics of overweight and obese patients with or without PCOS [21, 22]. In an early study in 33 overweight patients with PCOS, weight loss achieved with a low-calorie diet along with exercise resulted in resumption of regular cycles in 18 patients, spontaneous ovulation in 15 patients and spontaneous pregnancy in 10 patients [19]. In a more recent larger study in 143 obese patients with PCOS, weight loss through lifestyle changes improved menstrual frequency [20]. It should be mentioned that there are no data on specific dietary intervention and exercise for PCOS. Lifestyle changes are better defined as behavior modifications and correction of inappropriate dietary habits. Weight loss occurs when energy consumption exceeds energy uptake. Exercise is an integral component of every weight control program. Even though limiting energy consumption with diet is a major driver of initial weight loss, regular exercise contributes to sustained weight loss and reduces the risk for weight regain. Lifestyle changes are an important therapeutic strategy for all overweight and obese patients with PCOS [21, 22].

It is well known that aging is associated with progressive weight gain of approximately 0.5–1.0 kg annually after the age of 30 years. Therefore, maintaining the same weight during aging is considered a success. Weight loss is divided into two phases. A substantial weight loss usually occurs during the first 6 months, and this period is followed by a second phase where it is difficult to achieve further weight loss. This represents a physiologic adaptation and is due to the reduction of energy expenditure (plateau phenomenon) that follows weight loss. The second part of weight loss, which is the most difficult one, aims at maintaining the initial weight loss. The longer the period (ideally, lifelong) that weight loss is sustained, the more effective is the intervention implemented in an obese patient.

The initial target in an obese patient should be a moderate weight loss, i.e. 5–10% of the initial bodyweight. This recommendation is based on the findings of several studies, which showed that moderate weight loss significantly reduces the risk for obesity-related diseases, including cardiovascular disease, T2DM, hypertension, dyslipidemia, osteoarthritis and sleep apnea syndrome [23]. In addition, weight loss increases pregnancy rates [21, 22].

Dietary Modification

The diet of an obese patient should be balanced, i.e. should be made up of 50% carbohydrates, 20% proteins and 30% fats. Fat intake should be made up of 10% saturated, 10% polyunsaturated and 10% monounsaturated fats. The general rule of weight loss is 0.5–1.0 kg weekly that translates into a weekly caloric deficit of 3,500–7,000 calories. Carbohydrate intake should not be limited excessively, as it happens in the popular Atkins diet, because it might lead to acidosis, water loss, dehydration, cholelithiasis and electrolyte disorders, which might lead to arrhythmias and sudden death. Moreover, low-calorie diets should not include less than 1,200 calories daily, because substantial caloric restriction might lead to rapid weight loss, but this loss is only temporary and weight regain, i.e. relapse, is the rule. The method of very-low-calorie diets, which is rarely used, included a daily intake of 0.8–1.0 g of proteins per kg of bodyweight, 45–50 g of carbohydrates and a small amount of essential fatty acids. Daily calorie intake did not exceed 680–715 calories. Even though very-low-calorie diet is effective, it cannot be implemented because of limited adherence. Weight regain occurs very rapidly and, because the energy expenditure is reduced substantially, there is no further weight loss after an initial fast weight loss [24].

Basic dietary principles should be followed. Calorie intake should be divided into several small meals during the day, i.e. breakfast, lunch, dinner and two to three smaller meals between the main meals. In addition, there should be a balance between the different food categories, and carbohydrates, proteins, fats and minerals should be consumed in the appropriate proportions.

On a personalized basis, it is necessary to determine the daily basal metabolism in calories based on age, height and bodyweight, using basal metabolic rate calculation equations. Afterwards, a low-calorie diet should be administered, based on the calculated basal metabolic rate, with a daily calorie deficit of approximately 500–1,000 calories. In order to calculate the daily calorie intake, the patient's daily energy consumption, based on physical activity, should also be considered.

Exercise

Exercise is defined as any kind of regular activity that increases heart rate above resting levels. This results in increased energy consumption that, when it is not compensated for by increased calorie intake leads to weight loss and is even more important for maintaining bodyweight [25]. Exercise includes for example brisk walking, stair climbing, running, cycling, aerobics and swimming. In addition, participating in group sports is also considered exercise. Nevertheless, current living and working conditions are mostly sedentary resulting in obesity. Therefore, women can use even more energy than with sports if they include more activities into everyday tasks.

Exercise guidelines issued by the American College of Sports Medicine and the American Heart Association in 2007 [26] recommend moderate-intensity aerobic (endurance) physical activity for a minimum of 30 min on 5 days each week or vigorous-intensity aerobic activity for a minimum of 20 min on 3 days each week or combinations of moderate- and vigorous-intensity activity for promoting and maintaining good health.

The World Health Organization recommends for weight loss moderate-intensity exercise 3–5 days per week, and ideally every day, including walking, swimming, housekeeping and gardening [27]. The duration of exercise should be 30–45 min per day or more than 150 min per week. This moderate-intensity exercise corresponds to approximately 150 calories of energy consumption per day.

Behavior Modification

The treating physician, during his consultations with the obese patient, should try to establish a friendly relationship and to set realistic targets of weight loss, and to have frequent contact with the patient. The medical advice to the obese patient regarding behavior modification should focus on patient self-monitoring (i.e. the patient should record on a daily basis the dietary intake and monitor the bodyweight) and daily exercise. In addition, the treating physician should reward the patient and acknowledge the efforts when weight loss is achieved. The physician should advise the patient to avoid dietary temptations and to focus on important messages. Moreover, the treating physician should offer psychological support to the patient because it has been shown that weight loss improves self-respect and decreases the prevalence of depression, whereas weight regain has the opposite effects [28]. Recently, in the management of obesity, several cognitive and behavioral models have been proposed, which originate from the theory of learning and aim at lifestyle changes. These educational models are particularly useful in obese patients with eating disorders, including bulimia nervosa and the episodic hyperphagia syndrome [29].

Pharmacologic Treatment for Weight Loss in PCOS

Lifestyle changes are ineffective because obese patients who lose weight relapse, thus regaining the lost bodyweight during the following 2–5 years. Therefore, supplementary pharmacological treatment for the management of obesity is frequently necessary, and has been shown to maintain more than 50% of the initial weight loss for a period of 2–4 years. However, after the cessation of pharmacological treatment, a gradual weight regain is observed.

Pharmacological treatment of obesity is recommended in obese patients with a body mass index (BMI) >30 or >27 with concomitant metabolic diseases, including T2DM, which might coexist with dyslipidemia or hypertension. The treatment goal is moderate weight loss, approximately 5–10% of initial bodyweight, because this has been shown to substantially improve fertility and the metabolic risk factors associated with obesity.

The antiobesity agents, depending on their mechanism of action, based on the equation of energy balance, are divided into two categories. The first includes centrally acting agents, which reduce food intake by decreasing appetite and inducing satiety or by increasing energy expenditure [30, 31]. Sibutramine, a centrally acting agent that was recently withdrawn from the market because of adverse cardiovascular effects, reduces bodyweight in patients with PCOS by 4.3% more than diet alone and improves insulin sensitivity and reduces circulating androgen levels [30, 31]. The second category includes agents with peripheral action, which decrease fat absorption [32, 33]. The main representative of this class is orlistat, which was shown to reduce bodyweight and also to reduce IR and hyperandrogenemia in patients with PCOS [32, 33].

Bariatric Surgery

Two small studies in severely obese patients with PCOS (n = 24 and 17, respectively; mean baseline BMI 50.0 ± 7.5 and 50.7 ± 7.1, respectively) reported a considerable weight loss (56.7 ± 21.2% and 41 ± 9 kg, respectively). In addition, the majority of patients achieved resolution of hirsutism, improvement in IR and restoration of normal menstrual cycles and ovulation; pregnancy was also reported in some patients [34, 35]. However, bariatric surgery for the management of PCOS should be recommended with great caution and only when specific strict criteria are fulfilled [36, 37].

Pharmacological Treatment for the Induction of Ovulation

Clomiphene Citrate

It has been suggested that clomiphene citrate represents first-line treatment for the induction of ovulation and pregnancy in anovulatory patients with PCOS. Treatment cost is low, the drug is convenient to use, adverse effects are relatively few and mild, and there are important clinical data on the effectiveness of the agent [38].

Clomiphene citrate acts by inhibiting the estrogen-negative feedback regulatory mechanism resulting in increased secretion of FSH and LH. The ensuing ovulation is the result of hormonal and morphologic changes in the developing follicles. Thus, treatment with clomiphene does not induce ovulation but restores and augments the sequence of events of normal menstrual cycle. However, it is not certain whether the efficacy of this agent is exclusively due to the change in the secretion of gonadotropin-releasing hormone (GnRH). The main factors that predict treatment outcome are obesity, hyperandrogenemia and patient's age [38–41]. More specifically, patients with a BMI <30 have higher live birth rates than obese patients [38–41]. In addition, clomiphene is less effective in older patients and in those with less pronounced hyperandrogenemia [38–41].

The starting dose of clomiphene is 50 mg per day. The agent is administered for 5 days, starting on the 2nd to 5th day of the menstrual cycle. The maximum recommended dose is 150 mg per day. If ovulation does not occur after the administration of 150 mg of clomiphene for 5 days, in two menstrual cycles, the patient is considered resistant to the agent and the treatment should be withdrawn.

The largest of the existing studies in women with PCOS suggested that monitoring women with ultrasound or with measurements of serum testosterone levels is not necessary for a successful outcome with clomiphene treatment [40]. The strategy of most large centers is to monitor patients during the first treatment cycle with sequential ultrasounds, since this allows the evaluation of the ovarian response to clomiphene, a finding useful to determine the clomiphene dose during the following treatment cycles. When this strategy is not feasible, a single ultrasound before the initiation of treatment depicts uterine and ovarian morphology.

Regarding the effectiveness of clomiphene, the largest and of higher quality trials report pregnancy rates up to 22% per cycle among women who achieve ovulation.

Treatment with clomiphene in women with PCOS is limited to six cycles. In order to administer clomiphene for longer periods, up to 12 cycles in total, the physician should discuss this option with the patient. The cumulative pregnancy rate, when six treatment cycles are administered, ranges between 50 and 60%.

Well-known adverse effects of clomiphene include flush, headache and visual blurring. Multiple pregnancy rates are lower than 10%, whereas ovarian hyperstimulation syndrome is rare. There is an anti-estrogenic effect on the endometrium and the cervical epithelium, but it is relatively weak.

Tamoxifen

Tamoxifen appears to be as effective as clomiphene in the induction of ovulation. However, this agent has not received an official indication for the induction of ovulation [42].

Aromatase Inhibitors

Letrozole appears to be as effective as clomiphene in the induction of ovulation, but, similarly to tamoxifen, has not received an official indication for the induction of ovulation. More studies are needed to establish the safety and efficacy of aromatase inhibitors [43].

Insulin Sensitizers

Insulin sensitizers, which improve tissue sensitivity to the actions of insulin in vivo, have been used in the management of T2DM for many years. The most commonly used agent of this class in clinical practice is metformin, a biguanide hypoglycemic agent, which is administered orally. Newer agents of the class are the thiazolidinediones, and the first member of this group was troglitazone. However, liver toxicity resulted in its withdrawal, but other members of this class are now available, including pioglitazone and rosiglitazone; however, both these agents have teratogenic effects. D-chiroinositol has also been used with limited success as an insulin sensitizer in patients with PCOS. However, data regarding this agent are very limited.

Metformin increases the peripheral action of insulin on glucose uptake, possibly by acting at a post-receptor level. In addition, it reduces the basal hepatic production of glucose. Moreover, metformin reduces lipolysis at the adipose tissue. Finally, metformin improves insulin sensitivity at the muscular tissue. Recent data suggest that a protein kinase, which is activated by adenosine-mono-phosphate, is implicated in all these mechanisms of action of metformin. The advantages of metformin include the lack of hyperinsulinemia, leading to lack of hypoglycemia (the agent has no effect on pancreatic β-cells) and the low cost.

Regarding ovulation induction, the most important observations were that the interval between treatment initiation and the first ovulation is significantly shorter with metformin than with placebo, that the regularity of the menstrual cycle is improved with metformin, and that these improvements are variable and moderate. Metformin monotherapy results in a mean of one additional ovulation during 5 months. More specifically, the increase was only one or at most two ovulations per 5 months. These results were observed with short-term administration of metformin (up to 6 months). The prolonged administration of this agent, provided that it would result in weight loss, might increase ovulation frequency, a hypothesis that requires further evaluation.

Spontaneous ovulation can occur within 3 months after the initiation of treatment with metformin. In several studies, the ovulation rate increases, without any change in bodyweight, an observation suggesting that the effect of metformin on ovulation is independent of weight loss.

It has been reported that monotherapy with metformin is less effective than clomiphene citrate in the induction of ovulation and pregnancy in patients with PCOS. It has also been reported that there is no benefit from adding metformin to clomiphene citrate in patients with PCOS except, potentially, patients with BMI >35 [38, 40]. In a recent study, a theoretical decision analysis model was applied to compare the effectiveness of clomiphene citrate monotherapy, metformin monotherapy, clomiphene plus metformin combination therapy and placebo for the induction of pregnancy and live birth in patients with PCOS [44]. The model was applied to a theoretical population of 10,000 patients with PCOS. Pregnancy rates were determined according to existing data. It was also evaluated whether results varied depending on the different pregnancy rates across trials. This study showed that clomiphene citrate plus metformin combination therapy results in higher rates of live births compared with other treatments. The next most effective treatments were clomiphene citrate monotherapy, metformin monotherapy and placebo. The authors concluded that the combination of clomiphene citrate and metformin is the treatment of choice for achieving live births in patients with PCOS.

The decision whether to continue the administration of metformin during pregnancy in patients with PCOS and impaired glucose tolerance should be made by the treating physician after balancing the risks and benefits. However, it is emphasized that metformin is a class B agent, i.e. there are no indications, in either animals or humans, of a toxic effect on the fetus or teratogenesis. Finally, data from a recent randomized controlled trial, which compared metformin with insulin in the management of gestational diabetes, suggest that metformin is an alternative to insulin for the reduction of perinatal morbidity [45]. These data support a potential benefit of metformin as maintenance treatment in patients with PCOS during the pro-, peri- and postimplantation period, because of their increased risk for gestational diabetes [45].

Gonadotropins with or without GnRH Analogs

The recommended starting dose in the gonadotropin treatment protocols is 37.5–50 IU FSH per day [46]. The starting period of 14 days, at least during the first cycle, is less likely to lead to ovarian hyperstimulation, and the same applies to the small increases in FSH doses (up to 50%) compared with the initial or previous dose [47]. The duration of treatment with gonadotropins in general should not exceed six ovulatory cycles.

The two low-dose gonadotropin regimens that are most frequently used are the step-up and step-down FSH regimens. In the step-up regimen, if there is no follicular development on ultrasound, the FSH dose is increased. In contrast, if there is satisfactory development of a follicle, the FSH dose is not modified. In the step-down regimen, the FSH dose is reduced as soon as follicular development is observed on ultrasound. The low-dose FSH protocols are effective for the induction of ovulation in patients with PCOS, but the FSH dose should be adjusted with caution in order to avoid adverse effects. It is also necessary to closely monitor the ovarian response in order to reduce adverse effects and increase the effectiveness of the treatment. Before treatment initiation, strict cycle cessation criteria should be determined. Currently, it is not possible to eliminate the risk for multiple pregnancies or ovarian hyperstimulation syndrome.

Regarding the concomitant administration of GnRH analogs (agonists or antagonists), the substantial increase in the risk for ovarian hyperstimulation and multiple pregnancy, along with the additional cost and the lack of increase in pregnancy rates, do not justify its use for ovulation induction in patients with PCOS.

Laparoscopic Ovarian Drilling

Laparoscopic ovarian surgery (LOS) applies diathermy or laser for ovarian drilling aiming at restoring ovulation and achieving pregnancy. The main indication for LOS in patients with PCOS is resistance to clomiphene citrate [48]. LOS can achieve single ovulation without the risk for ovarian hyperstimulation or multiple pregnancies. Following LOS, regular monitoring of follicular development is not required. This method is an alternative option to gonadotropin administration in anovulatory patients with PCOS who are resistant to clomiphene citrate. LOS is particularly indicated in patients in whom regular monitoring with ultrasound is not feasible. With current technical advances, the intervention is completed in a single session. The risks of LOS are small and include laparoscopy per se, the development of adhesions and the destruction of normal ovarian tissue. The damage to the ovaries should be limited as much as possible. Irrigation with specific solvents might be useful for the reduction of risk for development of adhesions. Finally, LOS should be performed by adequately trained physicians and should not be applied for other indications except infertility.

Assisted Reproduction

IVF represents an important option for the management of patients with PCOS in whom other treatments have failed. The rate of multiple pregnancies can be reduced by transferring a small number of embryos. There is no consensus regarding the optimal ovarian stimulation protocol. There is a clear need for more randomized controlled trials comparing the stimulation protocols using GnRH agonists and GnRH antagonists. It has been reported that pregnancy rates with IVF are similar in patients with and without PCOS. This finding suggests that implantation is not affected by the presence of the syndrome [49]. The increased rate of aborted cycles in patients with PCOS is attributed to an inadequate or, more frequently, to excessive ovarian response leading to increased risk for ovarian hyperstimulation. It should be mentioned that the administration of metformin, in addition to its other beneficial effects on the induction of ovulation, in patients with PCOS, who have increased numbers of eligible follicles, reduces the risk for ovarian hyperstimulation syndrome. The mechanism implicated in this beneficial effect of metformin is unclear [50].

References

1 Nestler JE: Metformin for the treatment of the polycystic ovary syndrome. N Engl J Med 2008;358:47.

2 Legro RS: The genetics of obesity. Lessons for polycystic ovary syndrome. Ann N Y Acad Sci 2000;900:193.

3 Dunaif A, Graf M, Mandeli J, Laumas V, Dobrjansky A: Characterization of groups of hyperandrogenic women with acanthosis nigricans, impaired glucose tolerance, and/or hyperinsulinemia. J Clin Endocrinol Metab 1987;65:499.

4 Legro RS, Gnatuk CL, Kunselman AR, Dunaif A: Changes in glucose tolerance over time in women with polycystic ovary syndrome: a controlled study. J Clin Endocrinol Metab 2005;90:3236.

5 Rotterdam ESHRE/ASRM-Sponsored PCOS Consensus Workshop Group: Revised 2003 Consensus on Diagnostic Criteria and Long-Term Health Risks Related to Polycystic Ovary Syndrome. Fertil Steril 2004;81:19.

6 Franks S: Controversy in clinical endocrinology: diagnosis of polycystic ovarian syndrome: in defense of the Rotterdam criteria. J Clin Endocrinol Metab 2006;91:786.

7 Zawadski JK, Dunaif A: Diagnostic criteria for polycystic ovary syndrome: Towards a rational approach; in Dunaif A, Givens JR, Haseltine FP, Merriam GE (eds): Polycystic Ovary Syndrome. Current Issues in Endocrinology and Metabolism. Boston, Blackwell Scientific Publications, 1992, pp 377–384.

8 Azziz R, Carmina E, Dewailly D, Diamanti-Kandarakis E, Escobar-Morreale HF, Futterweit W, Janssen OE, Legro RS, Norman RJ, Taylor AE, Witchel SF: Task Force on the Phenotype of the Polycystic Ovary Syndrome of the Androgen Excess and PCOS Society: The Androgen Excess and PCOS Society criteria for the polycystic ovary syndrome: the complete task force report. Fertil Steril 2009;91:456.

9 Diamanti-Kandarakis E, Panidis D: Unravelling the phenotypic map of polycystic ovary syndrome (PCOS): a prospective study of 634 women with PCOS. Clin Endocrinol (Oxf) 2007;67:735.

10 Jonard S, Dewailly D: The follicular excess in polycystic ovaries, due to intra-ovarian hyperandrogenism, may be the main culprit for the follicular arrest. Hum Reprod Update 2004;10:107.

11 Jakimiuk AJ, Weitsman SR, Navab A, Magoffin DA: Luteinizing hormone receptor, steroidogenesis acute regulatory protein, and steroidogenic enzyme messenger ribonucleic acids are overexpressed in thecal and granulosa cells from polycystic ovaries. J Clin Endocrinol Metab 2001;86:1318.

12 Willis D, Mason H, Gilling-Smith C, Franks S: Modulation by insulin of follicle-stimulating hormone and luteinizing hormone actions in human granulose cells of normal and polycystic ovaries. J Clin Endocrinol Metab 1996;81:302.

13 Salih SM, Jamaluddin M, Salama SA, Fadl AA, Nagamani M, Al-Hendy A: Regulation of catechol o-methyltransferase expression in granulosa cells: a potential role for follicular arrest in polycystic ovary syndrome. Fertil Steril 2008;89(suppl 5):1414.

14 Dumesic DA, Schramm RD, Peterson E, Paprocki AM, Zhou R, Abbott DH: Impaired developmental competence of oocytes in adult prenatally androgenized female rhesus monkeys undergoing gonadotropin stimulation for in vitro fertilization. J Clin Endocrinol Metab 2002;87:1111.

15 Pigny P, Merlen E, Robert Y, Cortet-Rudelli C, Decanter C, Jonard S, Dewailly D: Elevated serum level of anti-mullerian hormone in patients with polycystic ovary syndrome: relationship to the ovarian follicle excess and to the follicular arrest. J Clin Endocrinol Metab 2003;88:5957.

16 Qiao J, Feng HL: Extra- and intra-ovarian factors in polycystic ovary syndrome: impact on oocyte maturation and embryo developmental competence. Hum Reprod Update 2011;17:17.

17 Cardozo E, Pavone ME, Hirshfeld-Cytron JE: Metabolic syndrome and oocyte quality. Trends Endocrinol Metab 2011;22:103.

18 Brewer CJ, Balen AH: The adverse effects of obesity on conception and implantation. Reproduction 2010;140:347.

19 Crosignani PG, Colombo M, Vegetti W, Somigliana E, Goccati A, Ragni G: Overweight and obese anovulatory patients with polycystic ovaries: parallel improvements in anthropometric indices, ovarian physiology and fertility rate induced by diet. Hum Reprod 2003;18:1928.

20 Tang T, Glanville J, Hayden CJ, White D, Barth JH, Balen AH: Combined lifestyle modification and metformin in obese patients with polycystic ovary syndrome. A randomized, placebo-controlled, double-blind multicentre study. Hum Reprod 2006;21:80.

21 Sastre ME, Prat MO, Checa MA, Carreras RC: Current trends in the treatment of polycystic ovary syndrome with desire for children. Ther Clin Risk Manag 2009;5:353.

22 Badawy A, Elnashar A: Treatment options for polycystic ovary syndrome. Int J Womens Health 2011;3:25.

23 Franz MJ, Vanwormer JJ, Crain AL, Boucher JL, Histon T, Caplan W, Bowman JD, Pronk NP: Weight-loss outcomes: a systematic review and meta-analysis of weight-loss clinical trials with a minimum 1-year follow-up. J Am Diet Assoc 2007; 107:1755.

24 Rössner S: Intermittent vs continuous VLCD therapy in obesity treatment. Int J Obes Relat Metab Disord 1998;22:190.

25 Votruba SB, Horvitz MA, Schoeller DA: The role of exercise in the treatment of obesity. Nutrition 2000; 16:179.

26 Haskell WL, Lee IM, Pate RR, Powell KE, Blair SN, Franklin BA, Macera CA, Heath GW, Thompson PD, Bauman A, American College of Sports Medicine, American Heart Association: Physical activity and public health: updated recommendation for adults from the American College of Sports Medicine and the American Heart Association. Circulation 2007;116:1081.

27 WHO: Technical Report 916 Diet, Nutrition and Prevention of Chronic Diseases 2003.

28 Schmidt U: Behavioral therapy, cognitive behavioral therapy and cognitive-analytic methods in treatment of anorexia. Psychother Psychosom Med Psychol 1997;47:316.

29 Spangler DL: Cognitive-behavioral therapy for bulimia nervosa: an illustration. J Clin Psychol 1999; 55:699.

30 Florakis D, Diamanti-Kandarakis E, Katsikis I, Nassis GP, Karkanaki A, Georgopoulos N, Panidis D: Effect of hypocaloric diet plus sibutramine treatment on hormonal and metabolic features in overweight and obese women with polycystic ovary syndrome; a randomized, 24-week study. Int J Obes (Lond) 2008;32:692.

31 Lindholm A, Bixo M, Björn I, Wölner-Hanssen P, Eliasson M, Larsson A, Johnson O, Poromaa IS: Effect of sibutramine on weight reduction in women with polycystic ovary syndrome: a randomized, double-blind, placebo-controlled trial. Fertil Steril 2008;89:1221.

32 Panidis D, Farmakiotis D, Rousso D, Kourtis A, Katsikis I, Krassas G: Obesity, weight loss, and the polycystic ovary syndrome: effect of treatment with diet and orlistat for 24 weeks on insulin resistance and androgen levels. Fertil Steril 2008;89:899.

33 Diamanti-Kandarakis E, Katsikis I, Piperi C, Alexandraki K, Panidis D: Effect of long-term orlistat treatment on serum levels of advanced glycation end-products in women with polycystic ovary syndrome. Clin Endocrinol (Oxf) 2007; 66:103.

34 Eid GM, Cottam DR, Velcu LM, Mattar SG, Korytkowski MT, Gosman G, Hindi P, Schauer PR: Effective treatment of polycystic ovarian syndrome with Roux-en-Y gastric bypass. Surg Obes Relat Dis 2005;1:77.

35 Escobar-Morreale HF, Botella-Carretero JI, Alvarez-Blasco F, Sancho J, San Millán JL: The polycystic ovary syndrome associated with morbid obesity may resolve after weight loss induced by bariatric surgery. J Clin Endocrinol Metab 2005;90:6364.

36 NIH Conference: Gastrointestinal surgery for severe obesity. Consensus Development Conference Panel. Ann Intern Med 1991;115:956.

37 Mechanick JI, Kushner RF, Sugerman HJ, Gonzalez-Campoy JM, Collazo-Clavell ML, Guven S, Spitz AF, Apovian CM, Livingston EH, Brolin R, Sarwer DB, Anderson WA, Dixon J: American Association of Clinical Endocrinologists, the Obesity Society, and American Society for Metabolic & Bariatric Surgery Medical Guidelines for Clinical Practice for the Perioperative Nutritional, Metabolic, and Nonsurgical Support of the Bariatric Surgery Patient. Endocr Pract 2008;14(suppl 1):1.

38 Thessaloniki ESHRE/ASRM-Sponsored PCOS Consensus Workshop Group: Consensus on infertility treatment related to polycystic ovary syndrome. Fertil Steril 2008;89:505.

39 Panidis D, Farmakiotis D: Treatment of infertility in the polycystic ovary syndrome. N Engl J Med 2007; 356:1999.

40 Legro RS, Barnhart HX, Schlaff WD, Carr BR, Diamond MP, Carson SA, Steinkampf MP, Coutifaris C, Mcgovern PG, Cataldo NA, Gosman GG, Nestler JE, Giudice LC, Leppert PC, Myers ER, Cooperative Multicenter Reproductive Medicine Network: Clomiphene, metformin, or both for infertility in the polycystic ovary syndrome. N Engl J Med 2007; 356:551.

41 Imani B, Eijkemans MJ, te Velde ER, Habbema JD, Fauser BC: A nomogram to predict the probability of live birth after clomiphene citrate induction of ovulation in normogonadotropic oligoamenorrheic infertility. Fertil Steril 2002;77:91.

42 Steiner AZ, Terplan M, Paulson RJ: Comparison of tamoxifen and clomiphene citrate for ovulation induction: a meta-analysis. Hum Reprod 2005; 20: 1511.

43 Papanikolaou EG, Polyzos NP, Humaidan P, Pados G, Bosch E, Tournaye H, Tarlatzis B: Aromatase inhibitors in stimulated IVF cycles. Reprod Biol Endocrinol 2011;9:85.

44 Jungheim ES, Odibo AO: Fertility treatment in women with polycystic ovary syndrome: a decision analysis of different oral ovulation induction agents. Fertil Steril 2010;94:2659.

45 Rowan JA, Hague WM, Gao W, Battin MR, Moore MP, Mig Trial Investigators: Metformin versus insulin for the treatment of gestational diabetes. N Engl J Med 2008;358:2003.
46 Balasch J, Fábregues F, Creus M, Casamitjana R, Puerto B, Vanrell JA: Recombinant human follicle-stimulating hormone for ovulation induction in polycystic ovary syndrome: a prospective, randomized trial of two starting doses in a chronic low-dose step-up protocol. J Assist Reprod Genet 2000;17:561.
47 Dale O, Tanbo T, Lunde O, Abyholm T: Ovulation induction with low-dose follicle-stimulating hormone in women with the polycystic ovary syndrome. Acta Obstet Gynecol Scand 1993;72:43.
48 Poujade O, Gervaise A, Faivre E, Deffieux X, Fernandez H: Surgical management of infertility due to polycystic ovarian syndrome after failure of medical management. Eur J Obstet Gynecol Reprod Biol 2011;158:242.
49 Heijnen EM, Eijkemans MJ, Hughes EG, Laven JS, Macklon NS, Fauser BC: A meta-analysis of outcomes of conventional IVF in women with polycystic ovary syndrome. Hum Reprod Update 2006;12:13.
50 Palomba S, Falbo A, Carrillo L, Villani MT, Orio F, Russo T, Di Cello A, Cappiello F, Capasso S, Tolino A, Colao A, Mastrantonio P, La Sala GB, Zullo F, Cittadini E, The Metformin in High Responder Italian Group: Metformin reduces risk of ovarian hyperstimulation syndrome in patients with polycystic ovary syndrome during gonadotropin-stimulated in vitro fertilization cycles: a randomized, controlled trial. Fertil Steril 2011;96:1384.

Efstathios Papadakis, MD
Division of Endocrinology and Human Reproduction
Second Department of Obstetrics and Gynecology
Hippokration Hospital, Aristotle University of Thessaloniki
Konstantinoupoleos 49
GR–54642 Thessaloniki (Greece)
Tel. +30 2310892129, E-Mail stpapadakis@yahoo.com

Macut D, Pfeifer M, Yildiz BO, Diamanti-Kandarakis E (eds): Polycystic Ovary Syndrome. Novel Insights into Causes and Therapy. Front Horm Res. Basel, Karger, 2013, vol 40, pp 142–157

Endocrinopathies and Other Disorders Inducing a Polycystic Ovary Syndrome Phenotype

Krystallenia I. Alexandraki · Gregory A. Kaltsas

Department of Pathophysiology, National University of Athens, Athens, Greece

Abstract

Amongst the commonest endocrine symptoms encountered in premenopausal women are those related to excessive androgen secretion or action, along with menstrual irregularity. The vast majority of women presenting with such symptoms will be found to have the polycystic ovary syndrome (PCOS), a disorder characterized by specific clinical, endocrine and ultrasonographic features. PCOS is regarded as a state of 'functional hyperandrogenism', as no distinct source of autonomous androgen secretion is identified and is commonly associated with insulin resistance. This later feature may also be related to some long-term sequelae of the syndrome that are associated with metabolic abnormalities and excessive cardiovascular morbidity. Although PCOS in the short-term is regarded as a 'benign' disease, a proportion of patients may harbor other underlying disorders that can be life-threatening, requiring prompt diagnosis and treatment. Adrenal and ovarian androgen-secreting tumors, adrenal and ovarian steroidogenic deficiencies along with other medical or endocrine conditions, particularly in the presence of insulin resistance, can exhibit similar clinical, endocrine and/or ultrasonographic features to PCOS. Their early identification is based on the presence of distinct features and a high index of suspicion.

Symptoms and signs of hyperandrogenism, namely hirsutism and acne, and menstrual irregularity in the form of chronic anovulation are amongst the most common endocrine abnormalities found in premenopausal women [1, 2]. The vast majority of such women will be found to have the polycystic ovary syndrome (PCOS), a chronic disorder usually manifested from adolescence, characterized by distinct endocrine abnormalities and the presence of polycystic ovaries (PCO) on ovarian ultrasonography [1, 2]. Although PCO can be found in 21–23% of premenopausal women, approximately 7% will develop the full clinical and endocrinological manifestations of PCOS [3]. This implies that additional factors may also operate for the development of the syndrome, the most probable being hyperinsulinemia and insulin resistance (IR) [4]. Recently an International Consensus Group proposed that PCOS can be diagnosed when at least two of the following criteria are present: oligo-ovulation or anovulation (usually manifested as oligomenorrhea or amenorrhea), elevated circulating androgen levels (hyperandrogenism), and PCO as defined by ultrasonography [5]. It was also suggested by the same group that the diagnosis of PCOS can be made with certainty when other medical conditions exhibiting similar clinical endocrine and ultrasonographic manifestations have been excluded [2, 4, 5].

Current understanding of the pathogenesis of PCOS suggests that it is a complex, multigenic disorder [4]. Genes that regulate the hypothalamo-pituitary-ovarian axis and those responsible for the development of IR appear to be related to the development of PCOS. Although alterations of gonadotropin secretion, particularly luteinizing hormone (LH), are implicated in the development of PCOS, disorders associated with hypersecretion of these hormones are extremely rare. In contrast, alterations of insulin secretion and/or action are found in many common disorders that are related to PCOS (table 1). Insulin, either alone or in association with LH, enhances androgen production from the ovaries while inhibiting hepatic synthesis of sex hormone-binding globulin (SHBG) from the liver; the net result of this effect is an increase in the biologically active androgens [2, 4]. This notion is further reinforced by the findings that hyperinsulinemia and IR are more prominent in women with PCOS and menstrual irregularity irrespective of the presence of obesity [4]. Excessive insulin levels correlate with the clinical severity of the syndrome and exert a stimulatory effect on the ovaries that remain sensitive to its action [6]. In addition, when obesity is present, IR is exacerbated further contributing to the worsening of the clinical phenotype [6]. It is therefore possible that hyperinsulinemia and IR may be implicated as an underlying pathogenic mechanism in several disorders associated with a PCOS-like phenotype [2] (table 1). In addition, a number of disorders associated with excessive androgen production from the adrenals and/or ovaries, or that affect steroid biosynthesis, secretion, metabolism and/or action, may exhibit similar to the PCOS clinical, endocrine and/or ultrasonographic features [2] (table 1).

Although PCOS remains the underlying diagnosis when such alternate diseases are excluded, the extent to which patients presenting with a PCOS phenotype should be investigated for other diseases has not yet been defined [2, 7]. It is estimated that the prevalence of disorders other than PCOS in women presenting with such symptoms is less than 7%; however, a number of them can cause considerable morbidity and/or even can be life-threatening [2, 8]. It is therefore important to be aware of the distinct features that these diseases may harbor to be able to identify them promptly.

Table 1. Disorders associated with the PCOS phenotype

Adrenal hyperandrogenism
Congenital adrenal hyperplasia
Adrenal androgen-producing tumors (adenomas, carcinomas)
Abnormal cortisol action and/or metabolism
Ovarian hyperandrogenism
Ovarian steroidogenic defects
Ovarian androgen-producing tumors
Hyperthecosis, luteoma
Ectopic LH secretion
Other endocrinopathies
Cushing's syndrome
Acromegaly
Hyperprolactinemia
Insulinoma
Ectopic LH secretion
Precocious puberty
Thyroid disorders
Syndromes of hyperinsulinemia and IR states
Lipoatrophic diabetes
Leprechaunism
Rabson-Mendenhall
Kahn types A and B IR
Diabetes mellitus type 2
Gestational diabetes mellitus
Obesity
Lipodystrophy
Other non-endocrine disorders
Epilepsy (?)
Intracranial hypertension
Drugs
Valproic acid
Growth hormone
Oxcarbazepine

Disorders Associated with a PCOS Phenotype

Disorders Associated with Abnormalities of Steroid Secretion, Metabolism and/or Action

Adrenal and Ovarian Androgen-Producing Tumors

Androgen-producing tumors, mostly adrenal carcinomas, and a wide variety of ovarian tumors can present with symptoms/signs of virilization (clitoromegaly, deepening of the voice, frontal balding, and muscle hypertrophy), hyperandrogenism

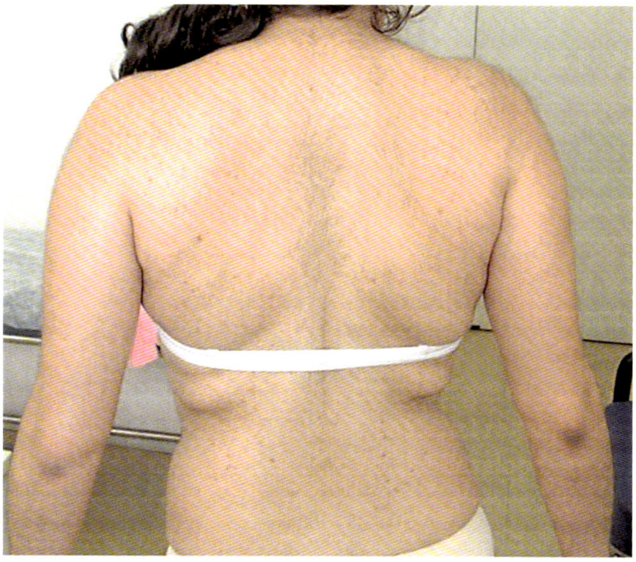

Fig. 1. Excessive hirsutism in a young woman who was found to have Cushing's syndrome secondary to ectopic adrenocorticotrophin secretion.

and chronic anovulation [7, 8] (fig. 1). Virilization seems to represent a distinctive feature for the presence of such tumors as it is extremely rare in women with PCOS, and when present it is usually mild. Adrenal carcinomas are large tumors that can hypersecrete testosterone or its precursors with or without concomitant cortisol hypersecretion. Ovarian neoplasms can be of variable size secreting mainly testosterone, although rarely can also co-secrete various androgen precursors [9]. Occasionally, ovarian neoplasms of epithelial origin may produce factors stimulating steroidogenesis in a paracrine fashion. Sertoli-Leydig cell tumor is the commonest virilizing ovarian tumor that occurs during the second to fourth decade of life and may be gonadotropin responsive [9]. A number of other tumors that also simulate the PCOS, such as hilus cell tumors, benign cystic teratomas and adrenal rest tumors have also been described; these tumors occur more frequently in postmenopausal women [8]. Ovarian hyperthecosis (nests of luteinizing cells distributed throughout the ovarian stroma) can present with a similar picture and be associated with severe IR [8]. The ovaries are enlarged and of an extremely firm texture as a result of extensive and dense fibroblast growth; the absence of follicle formation provides a clear morphologic distinction from the PCOS ovary [8]. The majority of virilizing tumors present during the middle age with symptoms such as rapidly progressive androgenic alopecia, deepening of the voice, increased libido and a male body habitus. However, particular attention should be paid to the rare cases of slowly evolving tumors, which can be clinically indistinguishable from

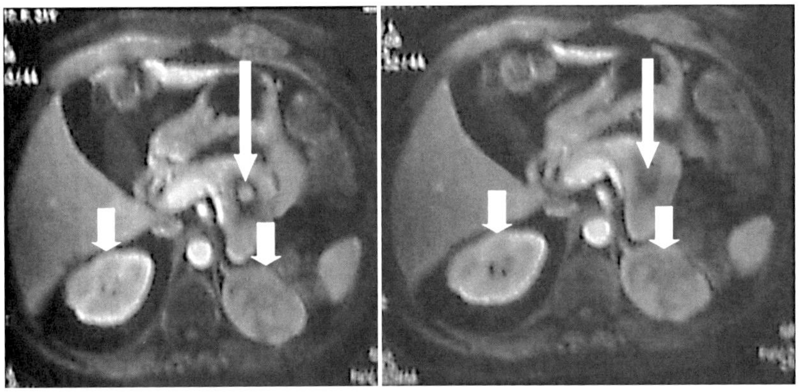

Fig. 2. T1-weighted MRI of the abdomen demonstrating bilateral adrenocortical carcinomas (short white arrows) and a pancreatic neuroendocrine tumor (long white arrow) in a 34-year-old woman with multiple endocrine neoplasia syndrome type who was initially diagnosed to suffer from PCOS.

PCOS [2, 7]. Although the majority of patients with tumors invariably have elevated androgen levels, only testosterone values >7 nmol/l (200 ng/dl) are highly suggestive of an androgen-secreting tumor [2, 7]. Occasionally, the documentation of an ovarian androgen-secreting tumor may be difficult as these tumors can be relatively small, eluding the detection with conventional imaging modalities [9]. Although in such cases bilateral adrenal and ovarian catheterization and sampling to document a gradient of an androgenic steroid has been employed, the detection rate remains relatively low [9]. Prompt diagnosis and management of these tumors are important, particularly in cases of adrenal carcinoma (fig. 2), as patients with localized disease exhibit a much more favorable prognosis compared to patients with more extensive disease [2].

Adrenal-Ovarian Steroidogenic Defects

Several enzymes of adrenal steroidogenesis can be affected, the most common being 21-hydroxylase (21-OH). Although classic congenital adrenal hyperplasia (CAH), which is mostly recognized at birth, is a potentially life-threatening condition, the nonclassic late-onset 21-OH deficiency or adult-onset form is the one that can mimic the features of PCOS [2, 8]. Late-onset 21-OH deficiency occurs in 1–5% of hyperandrogenic women, but has a wide ethnic variation [1]. Both classic and late-onset CAH, secondary to 21-OH, 11-hydroxylase or 3-β-hydroxysteroid dehydrogenase (3-β-OHD) deficiencies are associated with increased adrenocorticotropin (ACTH) secretion. The symptoms of adult-onset CAH develop due to the accumulation of serum 17-hydroxyprogesterone (17-OHPG), secondary to the block in cortisol biosynthesis, which results in androgen excess and PCOS [10]. It is of note that not all but 83% of adult and 76% of postmenarcheal patients with CAH have PCO [11]. Patients with CAH also have elevated insulin levels and are insulin-resistant probably due to the underlying hyperandrogenism [10]. The presence of IR enhances further adrenal and ovarian androgen production, probably contributing to the development of PCO, PCOS and the metabolic syndrome (hyperinsulinemia, increased triglycerides, reduced HDL levels, and impaired glucose tolerance) and its complications [10]. Adrenal and ovarian 3-β-OHD deficiency is extremely rare, and only a few cases of ovarian 17-ketosteroid reductase and aromatase deficiency have been described.

Premature adrenarche is a further condition associated with altered adrenal steroid secretion, characterized by the onset of pubic hair before the age of 8 years with no evidence of true puberty or adrenal dysfunction that can mimic PCOS [12]. Girls with premature adrenarche have elevated adrenal androgen levels secondary to ACTH stimulation, and an increased prevalence of PCO, and/or PCOS [12]. Similarly, girls with untreated central precocious puberty, initiation of puberty before the age of 8 years and therefore exposition to an increased androgenic load, have large-volume ovaries and a greater than expected prevalence of PCO, which persists even after standard treatment with GnRH analogues and growth hormone (GH) [2].

Alterations of Glucocorticoid Action Metabolism

Glucocorticoid Resistance States

Glucocorticoid resistance is a relatively rare condition that results from the partial inability of glucocorticoids to exert their effects on target tissues leading to excessive secretion of adrenal androgens secondary to a compensatory increase in circulating pituitary ACTH levels [12]. In women, excessive androgen levels can result in acne, hirsutism, menstrual irregularity, oligoanovulation and infertility, therefore mimicking the PCOS phenotype. Although the exact prevalence of PCO and/or PCOS in this group of patients has never been assessed, it is considered to be very rare [7]. The hallmark for this diagnosis is elevated cortisol and ACTH levels in the absence of any features suggestive of Cushing's syndrome (CS). However, the normal circadian rhythm of cortisol secretion is maintained, albeit at a higher level of secretion, besides the inability of dexamethasone administration to induce adequate cortisol suppression. The degree of tissue resistance can vary and as these patients maintain their sensitivity to mineralocorticoid receptors, arterial hypertension may occasionally be present secondary to the stimulatory effect of ACTH on zona glomerulosa steroid output.

States of Altered Glucocorticoid Metabolism

Alterations of enzymatic pathways involved in cortisol metabolism are associated with increased ACTH secretion which leads to increased androgen secretion, mainly from the adrenals. Rare enzymatic defects, such as deficiency of 11-oxo-reductase, which converts inactive cortisone (E) to cortisol (F), are associated with enhanced cortisol metabolism, compensatory ACTH hypersecretion and hyperandrogenism. Overactivity of 5α-reductase, which is involved in both cortisol and testosterone metabolism, increases cortisol breakdown and causes subsequent ACTH hypersecretion and hyperandrogenism while converting testosterone to more active metabolites, such as dehydrotestosterone, leading to hirsutism. However, both these conditions are considered very rare causes of PCOS [2, 7].

Glucocorticoid Excess (Cushing's Syndrome)
The great majority of women with CS, between 70 and 80%, develop menstrual irregularity and symptoms/signs of hyperandrogenism [13]. These findings along with truncal obesity and acne may suggest the diagnosis of PCOS, but the co-presence of specific symptoms such as bruising, thinning of the skin and proximal myopathy are more indicative of an underlying glucocorticoid excess [14]. However, in mild cases of CS these symptoms/signs may be absent or subtle and not easily recognized. In patients with CS and menstrual irregularity, serum cortisol levels are elevated, whereas androgen levels are relatively normal, suggesting that the menstrual irregularity may be directly related to the degree of hypercortisolemia [13]. PCO were also found in 46% of patients with CS, while all patients had low SHBG levels, presumably as a consequence of hypercortisolism-induced IR and hyperinsulinemia; in these patients, menstrual irregularity correlated with the degree of hypercortisolism [2, 13]. This hormonal profile could account for the development of hirsutism in patients with CS, even in the presence of normal androgen levels, due to an increase in androgen bioavailability [2, 13]. Based on these findings, it is prudent to speculate that when cortisol levels are moderately elevated, gonadotropin secretion is still preserved maintaining ovarian steroid output. This could lead to menstrual irregularity and the development of a PCOS phenotype in the presence of an estradiol-sufficient state [13]. However, when cortisol concentration is higher than a critical level, a state of hypogonadotropic hypogonadism develops associated with estrogen deficiency [2, 14]. In this situation, the presence of PCO morphology and/or PCOS phenotype could be attributed to the gonadotropic effect that insulin exerts on ovarian function and steroid output [13].

Besides the presence of a characteristic phenotype, another feature that could distinguish women with CS from those with PCOS is bone mineral density (BMD) status [14, 15]. Women with CS, even when diagnosed in subtle forms, have universally decreased BMD as a result of the hypercortisolism, whereas BMD is preserved in women with PCOS. Although in its full-blown phenotype the diagnosis is easily made based on increased urinary free cortisol (UFC) levels, subtle cases may be difficult to diagnose. In such cases, UFC levels can be normal, and the diagnosis is based on the presence of abnormal cortisol secretion pattern characterized by loss of circadian rhythm of cortisol secretion, and failure of cortisol suppression with dexamethasone administration [14].

Endocrine Disorders Associated with Alteration of Androgen Secretion, Bioavailability and/or Insulin Resistance

Hyperprolactinemia
Menstrual irregularity with or without galactorrhea in the presence of an estrogen-deficient state is amongst the commonest symptoms in patients presenting with hyperprolactinemia [1, 2]. In addition, hirsutism, seborrhea, increased androgen levels, particularly serum dehydroepiandrosterone sulfate (DHEAS), and PCO have also been described in such patients [1]. In women with hyperprolactinemia, the prevalence of hirsutism and PCO ranges between 50 and 67% [16], whereas hyperprolactinemia may perpetuate IR contributing further to the development of PCOS. A direct effect of elevated prolactin levels on adrenal steroidogenesis has also been speculated following the demonstration of high expression of prolactin receptor in the adrenal gland [4]. However, besides the presence of this evidence, there are currently no well-conducted prospective studies investigating the prevalence of PCO and/or PCOS in women with different causes of hyperprolactinemia [2].

Thyroid Dysfunction
Decreased SHBG, increased free testosterone levels and altered estradiol metabolism have been described in patients with hypothyroidism. It has been estimated that 36.5% of hypothyroid patients have PCO [2]. Precocious puberty and severe PCO have also been described in women with long-standing acquired hypothyroidism. However, there are no large-scale studies examining the impact of thyroid dysfunction on ovarian function and morphology and the development of PCOS. It is possible that hypothyroidism may enhance the PCOS phenotype, and there may be a relationship between insulin secretion, thyroid and ovarian function in patients with PCOS [2]. Hyperthyroidism has also been associated with increased SHBG and subnormal cortisol, free testosterone and DHEA levels along with PCO on ovarian ultrasonography [17]. However, it is not known whether these findings are related to thyroidal derangement per se and need to be verified by further studies.

Acromegaly
Hirsutism and menstrual irregularity is found in approximately 40–80% of patients with acromegaly [18]. It has recently been demonstrated that PCO are more common in women with active acromegaly, and this could be related to either GH or insulin growth factor-1 excess and/or the associated IR [19]. The majority of patients with acromegaly have large-sized tumors which either alone or with concomitant hyperprolactinemia can result in either complete or partial gonadotropin deficiency with low estrogen levels [18]. However, a minority of patients may present with or without menstrual irregularity and hirsutism in the presence of an estrogen-sufficient environment. In such patients, GH-induced IR is thought to be mainly responsible exerting a stimulatory effect on the ovary [2, 18]. The low serum SHBG

concentration found in these patients and the inverse association of SHBG with GH, even in estrogen-deficient patients, could explain the development of hirsutism in the presence of normal androgen levels [18]. In contrast, patients with small-size tumors maintain gonadotropin secretion and ovarian function and remain estrogen sufficient, thus exhibiting an endocrinological profile similar to that of PCOS. This state of hormonal excess can operate to affect steroid production, SHBG levels and ovarian function, and lead to the development of PCOS.

Less Common Endocrine Disorders Associated with PCOS

A few cases of ectopic LH secretion from pancreatic endocrine tumors presenting with menstrual irregularity and PCOS have recently been described [20]. Androgen levels were related to LH bioactivity and patients exhibited a PCOS-like phenotype [20]. Hyperandrogenism, menstrual irregularity and PCOS has also been described in patients with insulin-secreting tumors that resolved after the removal of the tumor [2]. It was hypothesized that insulin directly affected androgen secretion either acting as a co-gonadotropin in patients with coexistent PCO or inducing PCOS per se as previously described [2, 4]. Although hyperinsulinemic hypoglycemia may develop noted in some patients after Roux-en-Y gastric bypass [21], there is currently no study specifically looking at the prevalence of PCO/PCOS secondary to bariatric surgery in such patients.

Disorders Associated with Hyperinsulinemia and Insulin Resistance

Syndromes of Severe Hyperinsulinemia and Insulin Resistance

The HAIR-AN syndrome stands for hyperandrogenism, IR, and acanthosis nigricans [2, 22]. The primary pathophysiological derangements are IR and hyperandrogenism, the acanthosis nigricans being an epiphenomenon of IR. In patients with HAIR-AN syndrome, the severity of IR is positively correlated with the degree and severity of hyperandrogenism. It is thought that hyperinsulinemia stimulates ovarian androgen production directly and hyperandrogenism itself produces IR. The relationship between IR and hyperandrogenism might explain the hyperandrogenemia seen in lipoatrophic diabetes, leprechaunism and Kahn types A and B IR, and the development of PCO even before puberty in women with hepatic glycogen storage diseases [2, 22].

Diabetes Mellitus Type 2

The prevalence of PCO in female patients of the reproductive age with type 2 diabetes mellitus (DM2) ranges between 68 and 82% [6]. More than 50% of these patients develop symptoms/signs of hyperandrogenism and menstrual irregularity. However, a recent prospective study found that PCO but not PCOS is a common finding in premenopausal women with DM2 as 62% patients were found to have normal ovaries, 34% had PCO, and only 4% PCOS [23]. The presence of a number of correlations between metabolic indices and reproductive features is in favor of an overall stimulatory effect of insulin to the ovary [6]. Although it has been suggested that patients with DM2 and PCOS are more insulin resistant than those without PCOS, this has not been reproduced in all studies. It is probable that the mechanism of IR in patients with PCOS is different to that found in patients with DM2, and hyperinsulinemia alone may be not sufficient in some cases for the development of this ovarian morphology that may be related to alterations of insulin function per se [2, 6].

Diabetes Mellitus Type 1

Although type 1 diabetes mellitus (DM1) is a disease characterized by complete abolition of endogenous insulin secretion, a certain degree of hyperinsulinism may exist, resulting from the relatively excessive insulin doses needed to maintain a strict metabolic control. This exogenous hyperinsulinism may lead to increased ovarian androgen secretion, and an increased prevalence of hyperandrogenic disorders in DM1 women. Hirsutism was present in 28.6 and 0.0% of women with and without DM1, respectively; biochemical hyperandrogenemia was present in 23.8 and 7.9% and PCO in 54.8 and 13.2% of these groups, respectively. Using the Rotterdam criteria the frequency of PCOS was 40.5 and 2.6% in women with and without DM1, respectively, and appeared to be associated with intensive insulin treatment [24]. A recent study that investigated the effects of insulin therapy on ovarian androgen production, hyperandrogenism and PCOS in 54 adolescents and young women with DM1 demonstrated that androgen levels were significantly increased in women with DM1 treated by intensive insulin therapy [25].

Gestational Diabetes Mellitus

Approximately 30–50% of women with gestational diabetes mellitus (GDM) have PCO [2, 26] and higher adrenal androgen secretion [26]. More recently, it was shown that among 188 pregnant women, 16% of women with GDM had PCOS compared to 6.3% of women without GDM [26]. Women with GDM and PCO morphology also have increased frequency of menstrual irregularity and ovarian androgen production. The relatively lower prevalence of PCO in GDM compared with DM2 probably relates to the fact that only women with proven fertility, thus exhibiting less severe forms of PCOS, develop GDM [2, 26]. As women with GDM and PCOS demonstrate abnormalities in insulin action and secretion and are at increased risk for developing DM2, the ultrasonographic appearance of PCO may be a predictive factor of altered glucose tolerance during and after pregnancy [2].

Obesity

Obesity modifies insulin sensitivity and gonadotropin secretory dynamics, and can be associated with hyperandrogenemia and amenorrhea, thereby mimicking PCOS [4]. Testosterone formation from androstenedione is increased, and because of the hyperinsulinemia-induced reduction of SHBG levels, the free androgen index is increased. A negative correlation between free testosterone and SHBG has been found particularly in upper body obesity, and this is associated with a high prevalence of PCOS symptoms in adulthood [2]. Typically, a central fat distribution is present with an increase in visceral fat as reflected by the increased waist circumference or the high waist-to-hip circumference ratio which both correlate with increased androgens, impaired glucose tolerance, impaired insulin secretion and action as well as dyslipidemia. Obesity by contributing to IR worsens the reproductive and metabolic sequelae of PCOS [4].

Lipodystrophy
Lipodystrophies are a heterogeneous group of disorders in which the primary defect is a generalized or partial absence of adipose tissue, which may be congenital or acquired in origin [27]. The severity of an unfavorable metabolic phenotype is attributed to hyperinsulinemia, and is proportional to the degree of adipose tissue loss. In women with lipodystrophy, hyperinsulinemia leads to increased androgen production from the ovaries, leading to PCOS. Acquired lipodystrophy is increasingly found among HIV-infected patients treated with highly active antiretroviral therapy (HAART) in particular [28]. Most of such patients gradually lose subcutaneous fat from the arms, legs and face, whereas other areas of the body are spared; some patients accumulate excess fat manifesting as buffalo hump, double chin, and increased waist circumference. The fat loss worsens with ongoing HAART (protease inhibitors and nucleoside reverse transcriptase inhibitors) therapy and does not reverse on discontinuation of treatment implicating a molecular mechanism responsible for the lipodystrophic phenotype of these drugs [28, 29].

Other Medical Disorders Associated with PCOS

It has been reported that women with epilepsy have a high prevalence of menstrual irregularity, hyperandrogenism and PCO [30]. Although this association was originally attributed to the effects of treatment with valproic acid, subsequent studies revealed that it was not related to any specific antiepileptic drugs, as it was also observed in drug-free patients. An association of idiopathic intracranial hypertension with PCOS has also been described [31].

Medications Associated with PCOS

Initial studies suggested that patients treated with valproic acid are at increased risk of developing PCO and PCOS compared to patients receiving other antiepileptic treatment but not in drug-free epileptic women [32]. Following some contradictory results [2], a recent meta-analysis revealed that when applying the newly criteria for PCOS, the incidence of PCOS in women with epilepsy treated with valproic acid is approximately 1.95-fold higher than in women treated with other medications. However, this difference is not apparent when the old NIH criteria are considered [32]. Treatment with GH has also been shown to increase the prevalence of PCO in children with precocious puberty who received this form of treatment. Although drugs such as diazoxide, phenytoin, cyclosporine, minoxidil, danazol, and anabolic and androgenic steroids have been associated with hirsutism and oxcarbazepine was associated with hyperandrogenemia and PCO, there is no firm evidence that they can induce the whole clinical picture of PCOS [2].

Clinical, Biochemical and Radiological Diagnostic Confirmation of Secondary Causes of PCOS

In most cases, the diagnosis of a disorder other than PCOS can be made clinically and substantiated with biochemical and when necessary radiological confirmation (table 2; fig. 3) [2, 8]. Clinical history of virilization and rapidly progressive symptoms are highly suggestive of the presence of an androgen-producing tumor [7]. It has been suggested that testosterone and DHEAS levels in excess of 200 ng/dl (7 nmol/l) and 7,000 ng/ml (19 μmol/l), respectively, can reliably distinguish such patients [7, 8]. However, cases of androgen-secreting tumors with androgen levels below these cutoff values have been described [2]. In order to identify patients harboring such tumors, the testosterone response during a 48-hour low-dose (2 mg) dexamethasone suppression test can be used [7]. Of 17 patients with androgen-secreting tumors investigated, none showed either a greater than 40% reduction or normalization of the previously elevated testosterone levels, whereas 88% of patients with PCOS showed such a response (100% sensitivity and 73% specificity in distinguishing virilizing tumors from PCOS) [7]. In cases of high clinical and biochemical suspicion of an androgen-producing tumor, computerized tomography imaging of the adrenals identifies adrenal tumors (fig. 2), and transvaginal ultrasonography or magnetic resonance imaging (MRI) ovarian tumors [7, 8]. In the very unusual cases where imaging studies are negative, venous catheterization and sampling to demonstrate a testosterone gradient can be of value, although this requires particular experience and expertise [9].

Late-onset CAH is clinically indistinguishable from PCOS, and the diagnosis is based on either elevated morning basal or stimulated early follicular 17-OHPG measurements [7]. A circulating level of 17-OHPG >2 ng/ml (6 nmol/l) obtained during the follicular phase warrants further evaluation by an ACTH stimulation test [7, 8, 33]. Because there is a wide variation in the prevalence of this disorder among different ethnicities, this should always be considered when patients from a high-risk population are evaluated. In cases of nonconclusive results, genetic analysis looking at particular mutations may provide important diagnostic information.

Patients with CS can be distinguished from patients with PCOS from the distinct clinical picture [14]. In cases with subtle disease without the typical clinical features of CS, measurement of UFC only may not suffice to distinguish them from patients with PCOS, who may also have mildly raised UFC. In such cases, the degree of cortisol

Table 2. Clinical, biochemical and ultrasonographic features in secondary causes of PCOS

Disease	Hirsutism	Anovulation	17-OHPG	E_2	Testo-sterone	Δ_4	DHEAS	LH	FSH	SHBG	IR	PCO %
CAH	+	+	↑↑	↑	↑	↑	↑	↑	→↓	→↓	↑	82
Virilizing adrenal tumors	+	+	↑	→↑	↑↑	↑	↑↑	$\underline{\rightarrow}$↑	→↓	→↓↑	→↑	25
Virilizing ovarian tumors	++	+	$\underline{\rightarrow}$	↑↑	↑↑	↑↑	↑	→↓	→↓	↑	→	>80
CS	+	+	$\underline{\rightarrow}$	→↓	→↑	→↑	→↓↑	→↓↑	→↓	↓	↑	46
Acromegaly	+	+	$\underline{\rightarrow}$	→↓	$\underline{\rightarrow}$	$\underline{\rightarrow}$	$\underline{\rightarrow}$	→↓↑	→↓	↓	↑	NK
Hyperpro-lactinemia	+	+	$\underline{\rightarrow}$	→↓	→↑	→	↑	→↓	→↓	→↑	→↑	50–67
Glucocorticoid resistance	+	+	↑	→↑	↑	↑	↑	→↓↑	→↓	→↑	→↓	NK
Altered cortisol metabolism	+	+	→	→↑	→↑	→↑	→↑	→↑	→↓	→↑	→↓	NK
Severe forms of IR	++	++	→	→	↑	↑	→↑	→↑	→	↓	↑↑	80–100
DM2	+	+	→	→	→↑	→↑	→	→↑	→	→↓	↑	68–82
GDM	–	–	↑	↑↑	→↑	→	→	↓	↓	↑↑	↑	30–50

Modified from Kaltsas et al. [2]. + = Present; ++ = present in severe form; – = absent; → = normal; ↑ = elevated; ↓ = decreased; CAH = Congenital adrenal hyperplasia; CS = Cushing's syndrome; IR = insulin resistance (lipoatrophic diabetes, leprechaunism, Rabson-Mendenhall, Kahn types A and B IR); DM2 = type 2 diabetes mellitus; GDM = Gestational diabetes mellitus; NK = not known; E_2 = estradiol; Δ_4 = androstendione; FSH = follicle-stimulating hormone; SHBG = sex hormone-binding globulin.

suppression following the administration of 1 mg of dexamethasone offers high sensitivity and specificity in identifying patients with CS, as they fail to obtain adequate cortisol suppression [14]. Biochemical evidence of hypercortisolism and hyperandrogenism without the clinical features of CS suggests the presence of glucocorticoid resistance and/or alterations of glucocorticoid metabolism [7, 12]. Although patients with glucocorticoid resistance fail to achieve adequate cortisol suppression with dexamethasone administration, they do retain normal cortisol circadian rhythm and may have a relevant family history. However, the final diagnosis may have to rely on genetic screening [12].

Clinical signs of acromegaly and hyperprolactinemia should be looked for, particularly when low SHBG but relatively normal androgen levels are found [2]. Prolactin and insulin growth factor-1 levels should be measured, and a GH suppression test

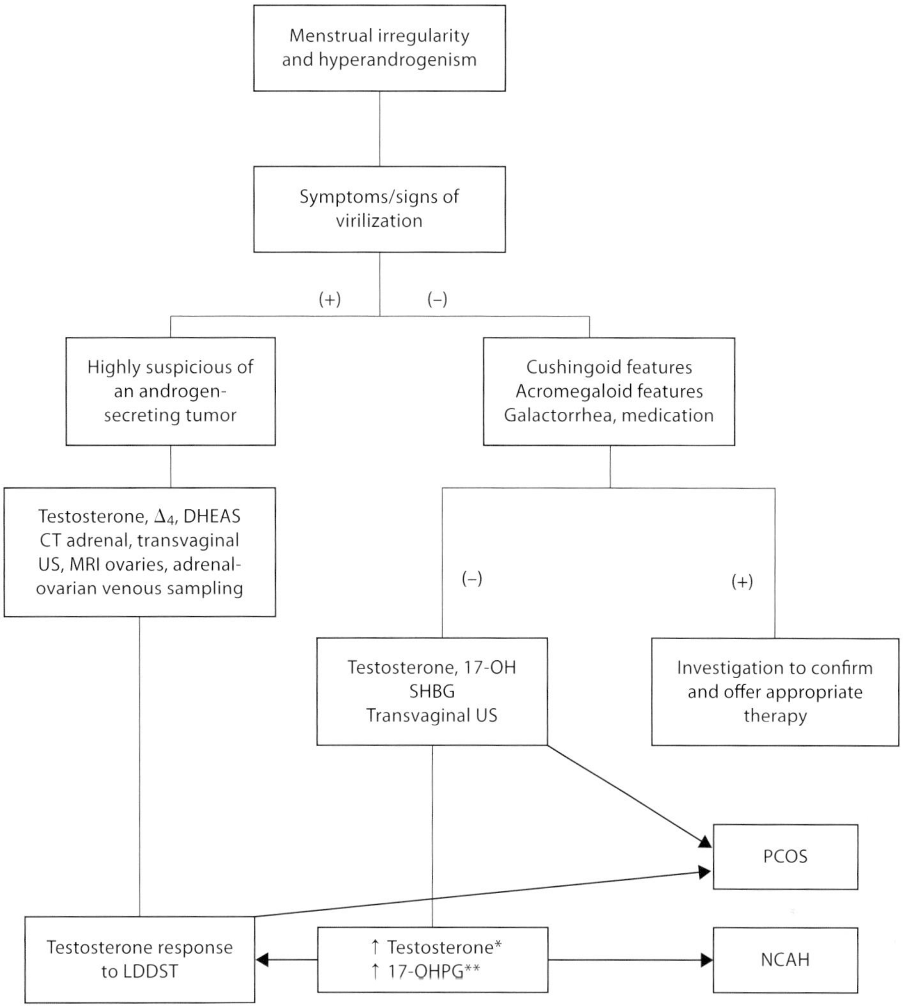

Fig. 3. Proposed investigational algorithm for the exclusion of secondary causes of PCOS. LDDST = Low-dose dexamethasone suppression test (0.5 mg every 6 h for 48 h); NCAH = nonclassic late-onset 21-OH deficiency or adult-onset CAH; SHBG = sex hormone-binding globulin; US = ultrasound. Testosterone response to LDDST means 40% reduction or normalization of serum testosterone following LDDST. Asterisk signifies testosterone levels 200 ng/dl, 7 nmol/l; double asterisk signifies 17-OHPG levels 2 ng/ml, 6 nmol/l.

performed, when indicated [2] (table 2). Pituitary MRI usually demonstrates the presence of a pituitary tumor in the majority of patients. Stigmata of IR and dyslipidemia (acanthosis nigricans and xanthomata) indicate the presence of severe IR, whereas an oral glucose tolerance test will confirm the diagnosis of DM2 or GDM in the relevant clinical setting. A detailed history can also reveal other underlying abnormalities or the intake of medications related to the development of PCOS.

Conclusions

The great majority of women with hyperandrogenism and chronic anovulation will be found to have PCOS. However, the clinical, endocrinological and ultrasonographic features are not specific to PCOS, as can be also found in other disorders, particularly in the presence of IR and hyperinsulinemia. A high index of suspicion is required in the relevant clinical setting to identify such cases and distinguish them from PCOS. This is particularly important in patients with androgen-secreting tumors and/or systemic disorders which need to be diagnosed and treated promptly.

References

1 Balen AH, Conway GS, Kaltsas G, Techatrasak K, Manning PJ, West C, Jacobs HS: Polycystic ovary syndrome: the spectrum of the disorder in 1741 patients. Hum Reprod 1995;10:2107–2111.

2 Kaltsas GA, Isidori AM, Besser GM, Grossman AB: Secondary forms of polycystic ovary syndrome. Trends Endocrinol Metab 2004;15:204–210.

3 Diamanti-Kandarakis E, Kouli CR, Bergiele AT, Filandra FA, Tsianateli TC, Spina GG, Zapanti ED, Bartzis MI: A survey of the polycystic ovary syndrome in the Greek island of Lesbos: hormonal and metabolic profile. J Clin Endocrinol Metab 1999;84:4006–4011.

4 Ehrmann DA: Polycystic ovary syndrome. N Engl J Med 2005;352:1223–1236.

5 Revised 2003 consensus on diagnostic criteria and long-term health risks related to polycystic ovary syndrome (PCOS). Hum Reprod 2004;19:41–47.

6 Conn JJ, Jacobs HS, Conway GS: The prevalence of polycystic ovaries in women with type 2 diabetes mellitus. Clin Endocrinol (Oxf) 2000;52:81–86.

7 Kaltsas GA, Isidori AM, Kola BP, Skelly RH, Chew SL, Jenkins PJ, Monson JP, Grossman AB, Besser GM: The value of the low-dose dexamethasone suppression test in the differential diagnosis of hyperandrogenism in women. J Clin Endocrinol Metab 2003;88:2634–2643.

8 Chang RJ: A practical approach to the diagnosis of polycystic ovary syndrome. Am J Obstet Gynecol 2004;191:713–717.

9 Kaltsas GA, Mukherjee JJ, Kola B, Isidori AM, Hanson JA, Dacie JE, Reznek R, Monson JP, Grossman AB: Is ovarian and adrenal venous catheterization and sampling helpful in the investigation of hyperandrogenic women? Clin Endocrinol (Oxf) 2003;59:34–43.

10 Charmandari E, Weise M, Bornstein SR, Eisenhofer G, Keil MF, Chrousos GP, Merke DP: Children with classic congenital adrenal hyperplasia have elevated serum leptin concentrations and insulin resistance: potential clinical implications. J Clin Endocrinol Metab 2002;87:2114–2120.

11 Hague WM, Adams J, Rodda C, Brook CG, de Bruyn R, Grant DB, Jacobs HS: The prevalence of polycystic ovaries in patients with congenital adrenal hyperplasia and their close relatives. Clin Endocrinol (Oxf) 1990;33:501–510.

12 Charmandari E, Kino T, Ichijo T, Chrousos GP: Generalized glucocorticoid resistance: clinical aspects, molecular mechanisms, and implications of a rare genetic disorder. J Clin Endocrinol Metab 2008;93:1563–1572.

13 Kaltsas GA, Korbonits M, Isidori AM, Webb JA, Trainer PJ, Monson JP, Besser GM, Grossman AB: How common are polycystic ovaries and the polycystic ovarian syndrome in women with Cushing's syndrome? Clin Endocrinol (Oxf) 2000;53:493–500.

14 Newell-Price J, Bertagna X, Grossman AB, Nieman LK: Cushing's syndrome. Lancet 2006;367:1605–1617.

15 Good C, Tulchinsky M, Mauger D, Demers LM, Legro RS: Bone mineral density and body composition in lean women with polycystic ovary syndrome. Fertil Steril 1999;72:21–25.

16 Isik AZ, Gulekli B, Zorlu CG, Ergin T, Gokmen O: Endocrinological and clinical analysis of hyperprolactinemic patients with and without ultrasonically diagnosed polycystic ovarian changes. Gynecol Obstet Invest 1997;43:183–185.

17 Skjöldebrand Sparre L, Kollind M, Carlström K: Ovarian ultrasound and ovarian and adrenal hormones before and after treatment for hyperthyroidism. Gynecol Obstet Invest 2002;54:50–55.

18 Kaltsas GA, Mukherjee JJ, Jenkins PJ, Satta MA, Islam N, Monson JP, Besser GM, Grossman AB: Menstrual irregularity in women with acromegaly. J Clin Endocrinol Metab 1999;84:2731–2735.
19 Kaltsas GA, Androulakis II, Tziveriotis K, Papadogias D, Tsikini A, Makras P, Dimitriou K, Stathopoulou A, Piaditis G: Polycystic ovaries and the polycystic ovary syndrome phenotype in women with active acromegaly. Clin Endocrinol (Oxf) 2007;67:917–922.
20 Piaditis G, Angellou A, Kontogeorgos G, Mazarakis N, Kounadi T, Kaltsas G, Vamvakidis K, Lloyd RV, Horvath E, Kovacs K: Ectopic bioactive luteinizing hormone secretion by a pancreatic endocrine tumor, manifested as luteinized granulosa-thecal cell tumor of the ovaries. J Clin Endocrinol Metab 2005;90:2097–2103.
21 Kellogg TA, Bantle JP, Leslie DB, Redmond JB, Slusarek B, Swan T, Buchwald H, Ikramuddin S: Postgastric bypass hyperinsulinemic hypoglycemia syndrome: characterization and response to a modified diet. Surg Obes Relat Dis 2008;4:492–499.
22 Tritos NA, Mantzoros CS: Clinical review 97: syndromes of severe insulin resistance. J Clin Endocrinol Metab 1998;83:3025–3030.
23 Kelestimur F, Unluhizarci K, Baybuga H, Atmaca H, Bayram F, Sahin Y: Prevalence of polycystic ovarian changes and polycystic ovary syndrome in premenopausal women with treated type 2 diabetes mellitus. Fertil Steril 2006;86:405–410.
24 Codner E, Soto N, Lopez P, Trejo L, Avila A, Eyzaguirre FC, Iniguez G, Cassorla F: Diagnostic criteria for polycystic ovary syndrome and ovarian morphology in women with type 1 diabetes mellitus. J Clin Endocrinol Metab 2006;91:2250–2256.
25 Bizzarri C, Benevento D, Ravà L, Patera IP, Schiaffini R, Ciampalini P, Giannone G, Cappa M: Ovarian hyperandrogenism in adolescents and young women with type I diabetes is primarily related to birth weight and body mass index. Fertil Steril 2011;96:1497–1502.
26 Koivunen RM, Juutinen J, Vauhkonen I, Morin-Papunen LC, Ruokonen A, Tapanainen JS: Metabolic and steroidogenic alterations related to increased frequency of polycystic ovaries in women with a history of gestational diabetes. J Clin Endocrinol Metab 2001;86:2591–2599.
27 Huang-Doran I, Sleigh A, Rochford JJ, O'Rahilly S, Savage DB: Lipodystrophy: metabolic insights from a rare disorder. J Endocrinol 2010;207:245–255.
28 Garg A: Clinical review: lipodystrophies: genetic and acquired body fat disorders. J Clin Endocrinol Metab 2011;96:3313–3325.
29 Viganò A, Manzoni P, Riva S, Brambilla P, Ferrazzi E, Marzi MM: Hyperinsulinemia induced by highly active antiretroviral therapy in an adolescent with polycystic ovary syndrome who was infected with human immunodeficiency virus. Fertil Steril 2003;79:422–423.
30 Meo R, Bilo L: Polycystic ovary syndrome and epilepsy: a review of the evidence. Drugs 2003;63:1185–1227.
31 Glueck CJ, Iyengar S, Goldenberg N, Smith LS, Wang P: Idiopathic intracranial hypertension: associations with coagulation disorders and polycystic-ovary syndrome. J Lab Clin Med 2003;142:35–45.
32 Hu X, Wang J, Dong W, Fang Q, Hu L, Liu C: A meta-analysis of polycystic ovary syndrome in women taking valproate for epilepsy. Epilepsy Res 2011;97:73–82.
33 Speiser PW, Azziz R, Baskin LS, Ghizzoni L, Hensle TW, Merke DP, Meyer-Bahlburg HF, Miller WL, Montori VM, Oberfield SE, Ritzen M, White PC, Endocrine Society: Congenital adrenal hyperplasia due to steroid 21-hydroxylase deficiency: an Endocrine Society clinical practice guideline. J Clin Endocrinol Metab 2010;95:4133–4160.

Gregory A. Kaltsas, MD, FRCP
Department of Pathophysiology, National University of Athens
Mikras Asias 75
GR–11527 Athens (Greece)
Tel. +30 210 7462513, E-Mail gkaltsas@endo.gr

Macut D, Pfeifer M, Yildiz BO, Diamanti-Kandarakis E (eds): Polycystic Ovary Syndrome. Novel Insights into Causes and Therapy. Front Horm Res. Basel, Karger, 2013, vol 40, pp 158–170

Non-Classic Adrenal Hyperplasia due to the Deficiency of 21-Hydroxylase and Its Relation to Polycystic Ovarian Syndrome

Duarte Pignatelli

Department of Endocrinology, Hospital S João, and IPATIMUP Institute of Research, Universidade do Porto, Porto, Portugal

Abstract

Non-classic adrenal hyperplasia (NCAH) is a disease in which a partial deficiency of the steroidogenic enzyme 21-hydroxylase produces mild to moderate hyperandrogenemia, hirsutism, polycystic ovaries, oligomenorrhea or amenorrhea, insulin resistance, male pattern baldness and subfertility. The resemblances between NCAH and polycystic ovary syndrome (PCOS) are manifest, and a relation between the two has been sought by many authors trying to identify subtle alterations in the CYP21 gene transcription end-products as the cause or a contributing cause of PCOS. On the other hand, the differences that may differentiate these two diseases have also been the focus of research by many groups, searching for clinical markers that might help to distinguish the two conditions. Insulin resistance or the polycystic ovarian morphology once thought to be hallmarks of PCOS have been proven to exist also in NCAH. Obesity, not being a diagnostic criterion of either but being very prevalent in PCOS women is also present in many NCAH women, and hence is not helpful in the distinction between the two. And if it is a fact that women with NCAH have a higher prevalence of normal ovulation and lower likelihood of having an LH/FSH ratio >2 or polycystic ovaries, in comparison to PCOS, it is also true that even in those parameters overlap does exist. Besides 17-OH-progesterone, progesterone, androstenedione and testosterone are elevated in most NCAH cases, similarly to what occurs in PCOS patients. The only exception in fact is the level of 17-OH-progesterone and progesterone that are not significantly elevated in PCOS, at least not to the levels attained in NCAH. Our recommendation, thus, is that NCAH should be excluded in all women presenting with hirsutism, oligomenorrhea and infertility. A basal follicular phase 17-hydroxyprogesterone level should be used as a screening tool, regardless of the presence of polycystic ovaries or metabolic dysfunction; in the case of doubt, an ACTH stimulation test is recommended. Levels above 10 ng/ml (30 nmol/l), either basal or after stimulation should be considered as diagnostic of NCAH, and some of those patients, particularly the ones that are planning to conceive, should be genotyped, mainly with the purpose of genetic counseling. Treatment of NCAH women normally requires the use of the same anti-androgenic weapons as PCOS but some may benefit from the administration of small doses of glucocorticoids. Curiously, some studies have demonstrated that PCOS cases too may benefit from the administration of glucocorticoids.

Androgen excess affects a significant number of women (approximately 10%, according to Azziz et al. [1]). Symptoms of androgen excess include hirsutism, alopecia, acne, ovulatory dysfunction, and in extreme cases, virilization.

Specific disorders resulting in development of hyperandrogenism include polycystic ovary syndrome (PCOS), 21-hydroxylase (21-OH)-deficient non-classic adrenal hyperplasia (NCAH), and androgen-secreting tumors. Distinguishing the first two disorders clinically has often proven to be difficult.

21-OH-deficient NCAH is one of the most common autosomal recessive disorders in humans, affecting 1 in 1,000–2,000 individuals but reaching 1% in some southern European countries and even 3–4% in Ashkenazi Jews [2, 3].

NCAH is diagnosed by the elevated levels of 17α-hydroxyprogesterone (17-OHP), and the disease can be confirmed by genotyping CYP21, in spite of the fact that not all mutations are identifiable in common genetic analyses. Clinical manifestations of this syndrome may include hirsutism, acne, alopecia, and ovulatory and menstrual dysfunction, but the degree of steroid 21-OH deficiency does not always correlate with the clinical manifestations with some cases being even asymptomatic [4].

PCOS is the most common cause of oligo-ovulation and consequently of infertility due to anovulation. It is also one of the most common endocrine disorders in women being implicated in the development of hyperandrogenic signs like hirsutism and acne. Besides, it was demonstrated to have metabolic implications resulting from its association with obesity and with insulin resistance (IR).

PCOS affects around 7% of the women in reproductive age [5]. Similarly to NCAH, the clinical manifestations of this syndrome include hirsutism as evidence of hyperandrogenism, and menstrual irregularities as evidence of ovulatory dysfunction. PCOS patients also frequently demonstrate IR, hyperinsulinemia, and polycystic ovarian morphology [1].

The pathogenesis of PCOS is probably the result of multiple factors, both genetic and environmental. It has been demonstrated to have an increased familial incidence, and in that context it probably is inherited as a complex genetic trait [5–9]. Inherited factors may involve genes regulating steroid production, androgen metabolism, the androgen receptor, folliculogenesis, insulin secretion, insulin action, obesity development, gonadotropins, among others. Numerous studies also support the involvement of adrenocortical steroidogenesis genes in PCOS pathogenesis.

As to the environment-related factors, stress and obesity are the two most likely contributors to the occurrence of PCOS.

The possibility that an adrenal steroidogenesis abnormality might play a role in the development of PCOS has long time attracted the attention of researchers. This could be either an enzymatic defect like 21-OH deficiency diverting steroid precursors to the production of adrenal androgens or an activation of the enzymes directly related to androgen production, notably CYP17.

Non-Classic Adrenal Hyperplasia Diagnosis along the Woman's Ageing

NCAH results from abnormalities in the gene CYP21 that encodes for the steroidogenic enzyme 21-OH. Since this is an autosomal recessive disease, affected patients have to carry mutations in both CYP21 alleles resulting in varying degrees of P450CYP21 dysfunction and clinically evident 21-OH deficiency. In NCAH patients, only a partial deficiency of the steroidogenic enzyme 21-OH exists, producing mild to moderate hyperandrogenemia appearing later than the classic forms of congenital adrenal hyperplasia (CAH) and not having the other strong symptoms that are observed in the classical, more severe forms, such as the deficient mineralocorticoid function (salt-losing forms), the early virilization/genital ambiguity or a significant short stature upon attainment of the adult age.

Girls affected by this disease may present with premature pubarche (PP) and acne. However, most studies refer that only 4–7% of the children with precocious pubarche have NCAH [10]. In some ethnicities, this has been reported to occur in as many as 30%.

Later, as they become adult women, some will develop hirsutism, oligomenorrhea or amenorrhea, male pattern baldness and subfertility. There is however a great variability of presenting symptoms inclusively, with some cases having no hirsutism or irregular menstruations and hence being identified accidentally. It is a fact that other genetic and environmental influences may occur and influence the final phenotype of each individual patient. The variations in androgen synthesis, secretion and metabolism as well as in the sensitivity to these hormones may significantly impact the expression of androgen excess. The expression of 5α-reductase in peripheral tissues together with the concentration and activity of androgen receptors greatly influences the final phenotype of each patient.

Among women with hirsutism, NCAH prevalence varies between 1 and 10% [11, 12]. Polycystic ovaries may also be observed in this disease, both in the classic and non-classic forms [13, 14], and this has been attributed to the alteration of gonadotropin release induced by the adrenal androgens or to direct effects of adrenal androgens on the ovaries. So, due to the overlap of symptoms, biochemical findings and ultrasound appearance, it is important to consider NCAH in every patient diagnosed with PCOS [14].

Overall, it is difficult to clinically distinguish PCOS from NCAH [13–15]. The possibility that differences in IR or hyperinsulinemia, or the presence of polycystic ovaries, might distinguish NCAH from PCOS among hirsute women has been sought, but this hypothesis was not confirmed [14]. IR, hyperinsulinism and polycystic ovaries were all observed in a significant percentage of NCAH patients. The conclusion was that due to the overlap of symptoms, biochemical findings and ultrasound appearance, it is important to consider NCAH in every patient diagnosed with PCOS [14].

Adrenal Androgens and PCOS

Both ovarian and adrenal androgens are produced in excess in PCOS. The principal source of androgens in PCOS is ovarian, but adrenal androgens are also significantly elevated both basally and in response to corticotropin stimulation. Adrenal androgens are identified by its major component DHEA-S since this is almost only of adrenal origin. Besides, it is the most abundant steroid in circulation, and its long half-life makes it very stable in the various phases of the ovarian cycle. DHEA-S is increased in at least 25% of PCOS women [16]. Other studies have reported even higher prevalence going up to 60%. DHEA, androstenedione and 17-OHP among others, have also been reported to be increased in these patients [17].

Adrenal androgens in excess may contribute to the development of PCOS. The concept of premature or exaggerated adrenarche that was developed by Samuel Yen in the 1980s was the first suggestion of that risk [18–20]. In the 1990s, McKenna and Cunningham [21] proposed that besides acting through a direct effect on the ovaries, adrenal androgens in excess could be peripherally converted into estrogens or more potent androgens, thus influencing gonadotropin secretion and consequently PCOS development. That process was shown to be reversible with glucocorticoid administration.

Pre- or peripubertal stress has been recognized to induce an exaggerated adrenarche with increased secretion of adrenal androgens and increased risk for PCOS.

And then, there is NCAH also supporting a role of adrenal androgens in inducing PCOS as this genetic disease may also have polycystic ovaries, elevated ovarian androgens and elevated LH [14, 22].

Adrenal hyperandrogenemia does not appear to result from 21-OH deficiency in most PCOS cases, although many studies have searched for CYP21 heterozygosity as an explanation for PCOS occurrence. It is also not known how polymorphisms in the other steroidogenic enzymes' genes may influence the occurrence of PCOS.

An alternative explanation is the observed increased activity of 17-OH that was reported in PCOS. Instead of an adrenal deficiency based in 21-OH, an adrenal hyperactivity sustained in 17-OH would be the cause of adrenal hyperandrogenism. A study observed an increase in urinary free cortisol in PCOS patients [23], and this could mean that the adrenal hyperactivity would not involve only the androgen pathway. However, other studies failed to observe increments in serum cortisol [24] and variation of cortisol and ACTH levels throughout the ovarian cycle [25]. Nevertheless, this may only mean that the metabolism of cortisol (for instance through 5α-reductase and 11β-hydroxysteroid dehydrogenase) is altered in PCOS. Studies have suggested an increased 5α-reductase [26–28] and a reduced 11β-HSD [29] in PCOS. The resulting possibility of developing cortisol deficiency would be compensated by an overall stimulation of steroidogenesis by ACTH that together with the increased activity of 17-OH would explain the hyperproduction of adrenal androgens.

Differentiating Non-Classic Adrenal Hyperplasia and PCOS

PCOS and 21-OH-deficient NCAH are different disorders which are difficult to distinguish clinically. A study aiming to determine whether women with PCOS would be distinguishable from NCAH women on the basis of having polycystic ovaries or evidence of metabolic dysfunction appeared recently [14]. Its results indicate that there are few clinical or biochemical differences between the NCAH and PCOS groups, particularly with lean PCOS women. NCAH patients were less likely to demonstrate anovulation, with more than 70% being eumenorrheic and ovulatory. Polycystic ovaries were present in only one quarter of women with NCAH as compared to 70–90% of PCOS patients (lean and obese, respectively), and maximum ovarian volume and follicle counts were significantly higher in both PCOS groups as compared to NCAH and controls.

In the study by Pall et al. [14], approximately 90% of women with PCOS, but only 17% of NCAH, had menstrual irregularities. The prevalence of menstrual irregularities in NCAH has been rather variable in previous studies (1.2–58%) but in all of them never as high as that of PCOS as defined by the NIH criteria. In the study by Pall et al. [14], the 10% of hirsute women diagnosed as PCOS that were clinically eumenorrheic were confirmed to be anovulatory by the concentration of luteal-phase progesterone. This also is consistent with earlier studies confirming that anovulation is a hallmark of PCOS (defined by NIH criteria).

Polycystic ovaries were observed in 80% of PCOS, and 24% of NCAH, but in only 4% of normal women.

While mean androstenedione and DHEAs levels were higher in NCAH, overlap with PCOS was significant. The mean LH/FSH ratio was similarly elevated in NCAH and lean PCOS women; however, the proportion of patients with an LH/FSH ratio >2 was significantly greater in lean and obese PCOS women compared to NCAH.

Obese women with PCOS had significantly greater degrees of IR and hyperinsulinemia, but the incidence and degree of metabolic abnormalities was similar between lean PCOS and NCAH women. The women included in that study, being of Portuguese origin, had a lower mean BMI than in several other studies examining PCOS, particularly those in the United States, where the prevalence of obesity is very high. That allowed the comparison of lean PCOS to NCAH patients. Diabetes mellitus was only found in obese women, although impaired glucose tolerance was found in all 3 androgen excess groups.

The most marked difference between NCAH and PCOS was the proportion of women with a basal 17-OHP level >2 ng/ml (6 nmol/l; 87% in NCAH vs. 25, 20 and 7% in lean and obese PCOS, and controls, respectively). The mild elevations in basal 17-OHP levels seen in both lean and obese PCOS in this study have been observed in other studies. Nevertheless, the fact that 87% of women with NCAH, but only 25% of lean PCOS, 20% of obese PCOS and 7% of controls had basal 17-OHP levels above 2 ng/ml (6 nmol/l) supports the use of follicular phase 17-OHP levels for screening (but certainly not for diagnosing) NCAH. The sensitivity of 2 ng/ml (6 nmol/l) as a cutoff level for NCAH was shown to be very high, in spite of the fact that 3/23 (13%) of women with NCAH in this study had basal levels below this value. These 3 cases were confirmed by genotypic analysis of CYP21.

CYP21A2 Gene

The disorders known as CAH are caused by mutations in the CYP21A2 gene, which encodes an adrenal microsomal cytochrome P-450 enzyme specific for steroid 21-hydroxylation (P-450c21). CYP21A2 is located in the highly polymorphic HLA complex region on chromosome 6p21.3, along with a pseudogene, CYP21A1P. Both CYP21A2 and CYP2A1P contain 10 exons. The genetic sequences of CYP21A2 and CYP2A1P are 98% identical in exons and approximately 96% identical in introns.

Over 95% of the mutations represent intergenic recombinations between CYP21A2 and CYP21A1P. Approximately 75% are mutations found in the pseudogene and are transferred to CYP21A2 during mitosis (gene conversion). About 20% are meiotic recombinations due to unequal crossing over during meiosis, which can produce a large variety of rearrangements depending on the breakpoints (gene duplications and gross gene deletions sometimes involving more than one gene). And finally, there are more than 100 additional mutations that account for the remaining 5% (reviewed in Speiser and White [30], and included in The Human Gene Mutation Database at the Institute of Medical Genetics in Cardiff, UK; http://www.hgmd.cf.ac.uk/ac/gene.php.geneCYP21A2).

The clinical manifestations of the disease are determined by the degree of the impaired enzymatic activity. Being an autosomal recessive disease, both alleles have to be affected, but mutations can be severe, moderate or mild according to the remaining enzymatic activity that results from their presence (0% for the severe mutations; 1–2% for the moderate and 30–50% for the mild). Large gene conversions, gene deletions, an 8-bp deletion in exon 3, F306-L307insT, Q318X and R356W are severe mutations. The splice mutation in the second intron (IVS2-12C/A > G) and the I172N represent moderate mutations. V281L and P30L represent mild mutations [reviewed in White and Speiser 31].

The phenotype will result from the less severely affected allele. Hence, the salt-wasting patients typically have severe mutations in both alleles, while simple virilizing patients will have severe/moderate or moderate/moderate, and non-classic patients can have severe/mild, moderate/mild or mild/mild genotypes. However, in about 10% of cases, the correlation between phenotype and genotype is not so clear. This is due to the fact that CYP21 alterations and 21-OH deficiency are a continuum between normality and the absolute impairment.

The Different Types of Congenital Adrenal Hyperplasia

CAH due to 21-OH deficiency is one of the most common autosomal recessive metabolic disorders. It has a carrier frequency of 1 in 60. Defects of the steroid 21-OH protein prevent the conversion of progesterone to deoxycorticosterone and 17-hydroxyprogesterone to 11-deoxycortisol, resulting in impaired aldosterone and cortisol synthesis, respectively. Cortisol deficiency leads to the loss of its negative feedback inhibition at the hypothalamic-pituitary level with the consequence of an increased ACTH secretion, which stimulates the accumulation of steroid precursors and their diversion to the androgen pathway resulting in androgen excess.

The level of androgen excess depends on the type of CAH being more intense in the classic forms of the disease than in NCAH. Measurements of unstimulated 17-OHP are often normal in this non-classical group, and so the diagnosis depends on the response to the ACTH stimulation test. This is done by administering 0.25 mg of synthetic ACTH (Synacthen®) intravenously and measuring 17-OHP and cortisol responses 30–60 min later. Other hormones can be measured simultaneously helping to identify other steroidogenic enzyme deficiencies. However, these comprise <5% of the enzymatic defects affecting the steroidogenic pathway. Progesterone, androstenedione and also testosterone are frequently also elevated in CYP21 deficiency. DHEA-s is not a good marker of this disease. Due to its long half-life, it does not respond to the ACTH test.

Deficiency of both cortisol and aldosterone synthesis results in the salt-wasting form of CAH, the most severe form of the disease. Androgens are elevated already in utero, which results in the development of ambiguous external genitalia in girls (virilization at birth).

The less severe form of classical CAH does not have salt loss, or this is only subclinical or manifested under strong stress situations. This is the simple virilizing form of CAH, where only cortisol synthesis is deficient and the manifestations result from androgen excess with various degrees of virilization of external genitalia in girls and prepubertal boys. Additionally, under stress conditions, adrenal insufficiency may appear.

Non-classic CAH (NCAH) does not have significant cortisol deficiency, and ACTH levels are usually not increased. Nevertheless, androgens are moderately to severely elevated, and in fact this disease is characterized primarily by signs of androgen excess such as PP, hirsutism, menstrual disturbances, and infertility.

In patients with CAH (classic and non-classic), it is generally accepted that there is a fairly good correlation (although not a complete one) between the intensity of the signs and symptoms and the mutations that are identified on genotyping the CYP21 gene. This led to the suspicion that since PCOS and NCAH are clinically similar, a state of heterozygosity of CYP21 mutations might explain the smaller elevations of 17-OHP, not attaining the cutoff levels necessary for diagnosing NCAH, that are observed in some patients in PCOS series. That way, subclinical NCAH could represent a significant percentage of the supposed cases of PCOS, for instance those with the strongest signs.

CYP21 Mutations Heterozygotic Carriers in PCOS

Many cases of NCAH are compound heterozygotes having two different CYP21A2 mutations. Genotyping women with NCAH is a difficult task due to the complexity of the gene, having a very homologous pseudogene, as well as due to the frequent existence of duplications, rearrangements and complex deletions many times involving more than the gene itself. Beyond the large deletions that cause this disease, more than 100 mutations have been described (in The Human Gene Mutation Database in Cardiff). So, in spite of the fact that the analysis of the 10 most frequent mutations will identify more than 90% of the mutated alleles [32] the detection of all carriers is difficult, and in most studies has certainly been incomplete.

Women that are heterozygotic carriers have only one affected allele. Their 17-OHP levels are only slightly elevated and overlapping with the levels of normal women. This means that heterozygosity should be suspected when a 17-OHP response to the ACTH stimulation test lies between 5 and 10 ng/ml (15 and 30 nmol/l) [33]. However, it was demonstrated that a normal 17-OHP response to ACTH does not exclude a carrier state for 21-OH [34]. Another study referred that the response of 17-OHP to ACTH was not predictive of having a CYP21 mutation carrier state [35].

An increased frequency of CYP21A2 heterozygosity was observed in cases of PP [36], and together with the observation that girls with PP are more prone to the later development of PCOS [19, 20] this favors the possibility that CYP21A2 heterozygosity might lead to the development of PCOS.

In adult PCOS, a study observed that ACTH-stimulated 17-OHP levels were above the cutoff limit in 20.8% of the cases, but, at the same time, only 9 of 19 patients genetically proven to be heterozygotes had elevated 17-OHP in response to ACTH [33].

As to the prevalence of CYP21A2 gene mutations carriers, Glintborg et al. [33] reported that this was 7.3% in women with PCOS and 6.3% in healthy controls. Witchel et al. [37] found CYP21A2 mutation carriers in 14.5% of women with PCOS and in 11.5% of control women.

So, for the moment, this similar prevalence of mutations in heterozygosity in PCOS and controls can only be taken as demonstrative that its contribution to the pathogenesis of PCOS is unproven.

Cardiovascular Risk in Non-Classic Adrenal Hyperplasia

Similarly to PCOS, NCAH patients have been associated with an increased prevalence of factors related to an elevated cardiovascular risk, namely obesity, IR and dyslipidemia [13, 38, 39]. In a vast study in the UK, metabolic abnormalities were confirmed to be very common in NCAH patients. These included obesity (41%), hypercholesterolemia (46%) and IR (29%) [40].

Nevertheless, evidence for the presence of cardiovascular disease or excess mortality in comparison with matched women without androgen excess syndromes continues to be inconclusive in PCOS [41] and even more in NCAH.

Obesity

Obesity has been looked upon either as a cause or a consequence of IR and hence a major contributor to the development of PCOS. Its contribution to cardiovascular risk is mediated by its influence on the increase in lipid levels, high blood pressure and inflammation. It is certainly not the cause of NCAH, but its consequences will probably be the same. In all of these women, it can occur due to the lifestyle modifications that affect modern societies contributing to obesity development in the general population. It can be determined genetically or through metabolic dysfunction such as that resulting from IR. It can also be induced by glucocorticoid treatment in patients that are treated that way. Another possibility would be an altered leptin axis [42]. More frequently than the occurrence of low levels of leptin, there would be a state of leptin resistance. Both glucocorticoids and insulin increase, while androgens decrease, leptin concentrations. In the future, it will be necessary to better define the role of the adipocytes in the occurrence of metabolic syndrome in NCAH.

Insulin Resistance

Both PCOS and NCAH are associated with IR [14, 40, 43–45]. Diabetes, however, does not seem to be more prevalent than in the general population [45]. It is a fact that the studies that have suggested that a percentage of CAH patients develop IR did not use the gold standard technique to measure insulin sensitivity (euglycemic hyperinsulinemic clamp method). In PCOS, IR occurs especially at the skeletal muscle level and only the synergic effect of obesity makes it present also at the hepatic level [46]. This specificity has not been studied in NCAH patients.

The resulting hyperinsulinemia seems to contribute to the increased production of androgens by the adrenal cortex [47] as well as the ovary. This is achieved by activating P450c17a (CYP17 mRNA and protein expression) and consequently augmenting the effect of the CYP21A deficiency that makes the steroidogenic precursors be diverted to the androgen production [48].

Besides obesity, hyperandrogenism and glucocorticoid treatment have been shown to induce IR in NCAH women. There are no studies assessing other risk factors such as CRP, homocysteine or TNFα. The same concerns the prevalence of carotid intima-media thickness. In fact, even the true occurrence of cardiovascular disease in NCAH has not been investigated adequately so far.

The conclusion that can be drawn is that long-term prospective studies are still needed to define cardiovascular risk in NCAH as well as PCOS. Nevertheless, risk assessment should be done in every patient, and lifestyle modifications aiming at a healthier living should be started precociously. This is based on the assumption that cardiovascular risk factors will predispose these patients to cardiovascular disease with aging.

Fertility in Non-Classic Adrenal Hyperplasia

Women with NCAH similarly to PCOS have reduced fertility. Several factors may contribute to this subfertility including anovulation due to increased levels of adrenal androgens or progesterone and in some cases secondary ovarian hyperandrogenism (PCOS) [49, 50]. Contrary to the classic forms, these women do not have genital ambiguity or an introitus that is inadequate to heterosexual intercourse. It is, nevertheless probable that even partial 21-OH deficiency affects endometrial receptivity, through the alteration of the hormonal microenvironment namely in relation to the elevated progesterone levels.

It must be stressed, however, that many patients conceive at a time when they do not even know they have the disease or conceive without glucocorticoid treatment when they are aware [50]. In some patients that fail to attain pregnancy, treatment with glucocorticoids may restore fertility.

In PCOS, menstrual irregularities and obesity are associated with decreased fertility rates [51], but this association was not studied in NCAH.

There is a significant risk of spontaneous abortion in NCAH patients (above 25%; in normal women this risk is inferior to 15%) [49, 50, 52]. Treatment with glucocorticoids seems to contribute to a decrease in that risk [50, 52].

Conclusion

In conclusion, the clinical differences between NCAH and PCOS are not clear-cut The same can be said about androgen levels. NCAH is a hyperandrogenic disease with androgen levels similar to obese PCOS but with a metabolic profile similar to lean women with PCOS. Nevertheless, some differences may be considered. As a group, women with PCOS are more likely to be oligo- or amenorrheic, have a higher prevalence of polycystic ovaries and LH/FSH ratios >2.

Subjects that are either lean or obese PCOS and NCAH groups demonstrate metabolic dysfunction. No major differences were observed in metabolic parameters when comparing lean PCOS with NCAH groups. In contrast, the obese PCOS group demonstrated a higher degree of metabolic dysfunction than the other groups. So, it is clear that the presence of metabolic abnormalities does not exclude the presence of NCAH, and it is possible that women with NCAH may have long-term metabolic and cardiovascular risks similar to women with PCOS [53]. Overall, screening using basal 17-OHP levels and acute ACTH stimulation testing remains essential to diagnose NCAH and distinguish it from PCOS.

References

1 Azziz R, Sanchez LA, Knochenhauer ES, Moran C, Lazenby J, Stephens KC, Taylor K, Boots LR: Androgen excess in women: experience with over 1000 consecutive patients. J Clin Endocrinol Metab 2004;89:453.

2 Azziz R, Dewailly D, Owerbach D: NCAH: current concepts. J Clin Endocrinol Metab 1994;78:810.

3 Speiser PW: Congenital adrenal hyperplasia owing to 21 hydroxylase deficiency. Endocrinol Metab North Am 2001;30:31.

4 Speiser PW, Knochenhauer ES, Dewailly D, Fruzzetti F, Marcondes JAM, Azziz R: A multicenter study of women with nonclassical congenital adrenal hyperplasia: relationship between genotype and phenotype. Mol Genet Metab 2000;71:527.

5 Kahsar-Miller MD, Nixon C, Boots LR, Go RC, Azziz R: Prevalence of polycystic ovary syndrome (PCOS) in first-degree relatives of patients with PCOS. Fertil Steril 2001;75:53–58.

6 Legro R, Driscoll D, Strauss J, Fox J, Dunaif A: Evidence for a genetic basis for hyper-adrogenemia in polycystic ovary syndrome. Proc Natl Acad Sci USA 1998;95:14956–14960.

7 Urbanek M, Legro RS, Driscoll DA, Azziz R, Ehrmann DA, Norman RJ, Strauss JF 3rd, Spielman RS, Dunaif A: Thirty-seven candidate genes for polycystic ovary syndrome: strongest evidence for linkage is with follistatin. Proc Natl Acad Sci USA 1999;96:8573–8578.

8 Yildiz BO, Yarali H, Oguz H, Bayraktar M: Glucose intolerance, insulin resistance, and hyperandrogenemia in first degree relatives of women with polycystic ovary syndrome. J Clin Endocrinol Metab 2003;88:2031–2036.

9 Ewens K, Stewart DR, Ankener W, Urbanek M, McAllister J, Chen C, Baig K, Parker S, Margulies EH, Legro RS, Dunaif A, Strauss JF 3rd, Spielman R: Family-based analysis of candidate genes for polycystic ovary syndrome. J Clin Endocrinol Metab 2010;95:2306–2315.

10 Armengaud JB, Charkaluk ML, Trivin C, Tardy V, Bréart G, Brauner R, Chalumeau M: Precocious pubarche: distinguishing late-onset congenital adrenal hyperplasia from premature adrenarche. J Clin Endocrinol Metab 2009;94:2835–2840.

11 Carmina E, Rosato F, Janni A, Rizzo M, Longo R: Extensive clinical experience: relative prevalence of different androgen excess disorders in 950 women referred because of clinical hyperandrogenism. J Clin Endocrinol Metab 2006;91:2–6.

12 Witchel SF, Azziz R: Congenital adrenal hyperplasia. J Pediatr Adolesc Gynecol 2011;24:116–126.

13 Robyr D, Llor J, Gaudin G, Schneider N: PCOS and CAH a different entity for comparable phenotypes? Rev Med Suisse 2007;3:116;1595–1596.

14 Pall M, Azziz R, Beires J, Pignatelli D: The phenotype of hirsute women: a comparison of polycystic ovary syndrome and 21-hydroxylase-deficient nonclassic adrenal hyperplasia. Fertil Steril 2010;94:684.

15 Moran C, Azziz R: 21-Hydroxylase deficient nonclassic adrenal hyperplasia: the great pretender. Semin Reprod Med 2003;21:295–300.

16 Kumar A, Woods KS, Bartolucci AA, Azziz R: Prevalence of adrenal androgen excess in patients with the polycystic ovary syndrome (PCOS). Clin Endocrinol (Oxf) 2005;62:644–649.

17 Moran C, Reyna R, Boots L, Azziz R: Adrenocortical hyperresponsiveness to ACTH in PCOS patients with adrenal androgen excess. Fertil Steril 2004;81:126–131.

18 Miller D, Emans SJ, Kohane I: Follow-up study of adolescent girls with a history of premature pubarche. J Adolesc Health 1996;18:301–305.

19 Ibanez L, Potau N, Zampolli M, Street ME, Carrascosa A: Girls diagnosed with premature pubarche show an exaggerated ovarian androgen synthesis from the early stages of puberty: evidence from gonadotropin-releasing hormone agonist testing. Fertil Steril 1997;67:849–855.

20 Meas T, Chevenne D, Thibaud E, Leger J, Cabrol S, Czernichow P, Levy-Marchal C: Endocrine consequences of premature pubarche in post-pubertal Caucasian girls. Clin Endocrinol (Oxf) 2002;57:101–106.

21 McKenna T, Cunningham S: Adrenal abnormalities in PCOS and the impact of their correction; in Dunaif A, Givens J, Haseltine F, Merriam G (eds): Polycystic Ovary Syndrome. Oxford, Blackwell Scientific Publications, 1992, pp 183–193.

22 Moran C, Azziz R, Carmina E, Dewailly D, Fruzzetti F, Ibanez L, Knochenhauer ES, Marcondes JA, Mendonca BB, Pignatelli D, Pugeat M, Rohmer V, Speiser PW, Witchel SF: 21-Hydroxylase-deficient nonclassic adrenal hyperplasia is a progressive disorder: a multicenter study. Am J Obstet Gynecol 2000;183:1468–1474.

23 Invitti C, Pecori Giraldi F, Dubini A, De Martin M, Cavagnini F: Increased urinary free cortisol and decreased serum corticosteroid-binding globulin in polycystic ovary syndrome. Acta Endocrinol (Copenh) 1991;125:28–32.

24 Vogeser M, Halser B, Baron A, Jacob K, Demant T: Corticosteroid-binding globulin and unbound serum cortisol in women with PCOS. Clin Biochem 2000;33:157–159.

25 Stewart PM, Penn R, Holder R, Parton A, Ratcliffe JG, London DR: The hypothalamo-pituitary-adrenal axis across the normal menstrual cycle and in polycystic ovary syndrome. Clin Endocrinol (Oxf) 1993;38:387–391.

26 Stewart PM, Shackleton CH, Beastall GH, Edwards CR: 5 alpha-reductase activity in polycystic ovary syndrome. Lancet 1990;335:431–433.

27 Chin D, Shackleton C, Prasad VK, Kohn B, David R, Imperato-McGinley J, Cohen H, McMahon DJ, Oberfield SE: Increased 5α-reductase and normal 11β-hydroxysteroid dehydrogenase metabolism of C19 and C21 steroids in a young population with polycystic ovarian syndrome. J Pediatr Endocrinol Metab 2000;13:253–259.

28 Fassnacht M, Schlenz N, Schneider SB, Wudy SA, Allolio B, Arlt W: Beyond adrenal and ovarian androgen generation: increased peripheral 5 alpha-reductase activity in women with polycystic ovary syndrome. J Clin Endocrinol Metab 2003;88:2760–2766.

29 Rodin A, Thakkar H, Taylor N, Clayton R: Hyperandrogenism in PCOS. Evidence of dysregulation of 11 beta-hydroxysteroid dehydrogenase. N Engl J Med 1994;330:460–465.

30 Speiser PW, White PC: Congenital adrenal hyperplasia. N Engl J Med 2003;349:776–788.

31 White P, Speiser P: Congenital adrenal hyperplasia due to 21-hydroxylase deficiency. Endocr Rev 2000;21:245–291.

32 Speiser P, Azziz R, Baskin L, Ghizzoni L, Hensle T, Merke D, Meyer-Bahlburg H, Miller W, Montori V, Oberfield S, Ritzen M, White P: Congenital adrenal hyperplasia due to 21-hydroxylase deficiency: an Endocrine Society Clinical Practice Guideline. J Clin Endocrinol Metab 2010;95:4133–4160.

33 Glintborg D, Hermann AP, Brusgaard K, Hangaard J, Hagen C, Andersen M: Significantly higher adrenocorticotropin-stimulated cortisol and 17-hydroxyprogesterone levels in 337 consecutive, premenopausal, Caucasian, hirsute patients compared with healthy controls. J Clin Endocrinol Metab 2005;90:1347–1353.

34 Witchel SF, Lee PA: Identification of heterozygotic carriers of 21-hydroxylase deficiency: sensitivity of ACTH stimulation tests. Am J Med Genet 1998; 76:337–342.

35 Escobar Morreale H, San Millan J, Smith R, Sanch J, Witchel S: The presence of the 21-hydroxylase deficiency carrier status in hirsute women: phenotype-genotype correlations. Fertil Steril 1999;72: 629–638.

36 Dacou-Voutetakis C, Dracopoulou M: High incidence of molecular defects of the CYP21A2 gene in patients with premature adrenarche. J Clin Endocrinol Metab 1999;84:1570–1574.

37 Witchel SF, Kahsar-Miller M, Aston CE, White C, Azziz R: Prevalence of CYP21 mutations and IRS1 variant among women with polycystic ovary syndrome and adrenal androgen excess. Fertil Steril 2005;83:371–375.

38 Kim MS, Merke DP: Cardiovascular disease risk in adult women with CAH due to 21-hydroxylase deficiency Semin Reprod Med 2008;27:316–321.

39 Wild RA, Rizzo M, Clifton S, Carmina E: Lipid levels in polycystic ovary syndrome: systematic review and meta-analysis. Fertil Steril 2011;95:1073–1079.

40 Arlt W, Willis DS, Wild SH, Krone N, Doherty EJ, Hahner S, Han TS, Carroll PV, Conway GS, Rees DA, Stimson RH, Walker BR, Connell JM, Ross RJ: United Kingdom Congenital Adrenal Hyperplasia Adult Study Executive (CaHASE). Health status of adults with congenital adrenal hyperplasia: a cohort study of 203 patients. J Clin Endocrinol Metab 2010;95:5110–5121.

41 Fauser B, Bouchard P: Uncertainty remains in women with PCOS regarding the increased incidence of cardiovascular disease later in life, despite the indisputable presence of multiple cardiovascular risk factors at a young age. J Clin Endocrinol Metab 2011;96:1–3.

42 Volkl TM, Simm D, Korner A, Rascher W, Kiess W, Kratzsch J, Dorr HG: Does an altered leptin axis play a role in obesity among children and adolescents with classical congenital adrenal hyperplasia due to 21-hydroxylase deficiency? Eur J Endocrinol 2009;160:239–247.

43 Saygili F, Oge A, Yilmaz C: Hyperinsulinemia and insulin insensitivity in women with NCAH due to 21-hydroxylase deficiency: the relationship between serum leptin levels and chronic hyperinsulinemia. Horm Res 2005;63:270–274.

44 Kroese JM, Mooij CF, van der Graaf M, Hermus AR, Tack CJ: Pioglitazone improves insulin resistance and decreases blood pressure in adult patients with congenital adrenal hyperplasia. Eur J Endocrinol 2009;161:887–894.

45 Speiser PW, Serrat J, New MI, et al: Insulin insensitivity in adrenal hyperplasia due to nonclassical steroid 21-hydroxylase deficiency. J Clin Endocrinol Metab 1992;75:1421–1424.

46 Sam S, Dunaif A: PCOS: syndrome XX? Trends Endocrinol Metab 2003;14:365–370.

47 Arslanian SA, Lewy V, Danadian K, Saad R: Metformin therapy in obese adolescents with polycystic ovary syndrome and impaired glucose tolerance: amelioration of exaggerated adrenal response to adrenocorticotropin with reduction of insulinemia/insulin resistance. J Clin Endocrinol Metab 2002;87:1555–1559.
48 Kelly S, McKenna T, Young L: Modulation of steroidogenic enzymes by orphan nuclear transcriptional regulation may control diverse production of cortisol and androgens in the human adrenal. J Endocrinol 2004;181:355–365.
49 Feldman S, Billaud L, Thalabard JC, Raux-Demay MC, Mowszowicz I, Kuttenn F, Mauvais-Jarvis P: Fertility in women with late-onset adrenal hyperplasia due to 21-hydroxylase deficiency. J Clin Endocrinol Metab 1992;74:635–639.
50 Moran C, Azziz R, Weintrob N, Witchel S, Rohmer V, Dewailly D, Marcondes J, Pugeat M, Speiser P, Pignatelli D, Mendonca B, Bachega T, Escobar-Morreale H, Carmina E, Fruzzetti F, Kelestimur F: Reproductive outcome of women with 21-hydroxylase-deficient nonclassic adrenal hyperplasia. J Clin Endocrinol Metab 2006;91:3451–3456.
51 Koivunen R, Pouta A, Franks S, Martikainen H, Sovio U, Hartikainen AL, McCarthy MI, Ruokonen A, Bloigu A, Järvelin MR, Morin-Papunen L: Fecundability and spontaneous abortions in women with self-reported oligo-amenorrhea and/or hirsutism: Northern Finland Birth Cohort 1966 Study. Hum Reprod 2008;23:2134–2139.
52 Bidet M, Bellanné-Chantelot C, Galand-Portier MB, Golmard JL, Tardy V, Morel Y, Clauin S, Coussieu C, Boudou P, Mowzowicz I, Bachelot A, Touraine P, Kuttenn F: Fertility in women with nonclassical congenital adrenal hyperplasia due to 21-hydroxylase deficiency. J Clin Endocrinol Metab 2010;95: 1182–1190.
53 Orio F, Vuolo L, Palomba S, Lombardi G, Colao A: Metabolic and cardiovascular consequences of polycystic ovary syndrome. Minerva Ginecol 2008;60: 39–51.

Duarte Pignatelli, MD, PhD
Department of Endocrinology, Hospital S João
Alameda Hernani Monteiro
PT–4200-319 Porto (Portugal)
Tel. +351 912880313, E-Mail dpignatelli@ipatimup.pt

Author Index

Subject Index